# An Atlas of

# Dentition
# in Childhood

## Orthodontic Diagnosis
## and Panoramic Radiology

Herman S. Duterloo, D.D.S., Ph.D.

Clinical Orthodontist
Maastricht
The Netherlands

Professor of Orthodontics
Former Chairman, Department of Orthodontics
University of Groningen
The Netherlands

Wolfe Publishing Ltd

To Sofia,
Eline, Victor, Maud,
Servaas,
Fridy,
and Jef
for their inspiration and encouragement.

Copyright © Herman S. Duterloo, 1991
Published by Wolfe Publishing Ltd, 1991
Printed by Hazell Books Ltd, Aylesbury, England
ISBN 0 7234 0951 X

A CIP catalogue record for this book is available from the British Library.

This book is one of the titles in the series of Wolfe Medical Atlases, a series that brings together the world's largest systematic published collection of diagnostic colour photographs.

For a full list of Atlases in the series, plus forthcoming titles and details of our surgical, dental and veterinary Atlases, please write to Wolfe Publishing Ltd, 2–16 Torrington Place, London WC1E 7LT, England.

WU 480

# Contents

# 1 Introduction

A brief review of historical aspects of panoramic X-rays; general advantages and disadvantages of the technique; its current status in clinical practice, and its potentials in research and practice. The second part briefly reviews the literature on the development of the human dentition. Recommendations are made for current literature study to enhance the understanding of the information provided in subsequent chapters. Indications for taking a panoramic X-ray during childhood are treated.

# 2 Working with the Panoramic X-ray Machine

The methods, techniques and procedures used to produce the illustrations. The X-ray machine, the craniostat and skeletal material are introduced; reconstructive procedures, marking techniques; handling of film material; patient positioning aspects. Because orthopantomography is frequently used in the mixed dentition period, a dry skull of that development stage is used.

# 3 Normal Anatomy of the Facial Region and Dentition

A systematic analysis of interpretation of panoramic X-rays, applied to five specific areas, described in detail, using one standard panoramic X-ray. The appearance of soft tissues is examined separately.

# 4 Normal Development of Teeth and Alveolar Bone

# 5 Developmental Chronology of the Dentition

The successive stages of dentitional development, shown in representative panoramic X-rays and drawings. Prenatal and development of deciduous dentition stages are excluded because panoramic X-rays of these stages are not feasible and only in exceptional cases are they of clinical value. Estimation of dental age is of utmost clinical importance, and adequate data are provided to be used in the clinic for estimations for individual patients.

# 6 Interpretation of Position of Permanent Teeth

Special reconstructions are used to demonstrate where and how to look on panoramic X-rays to evaluate the position of the teeth. These reconstructions help the clinician visualise the complex relative positions of a large number of closely packed three-dimensional objects—as the situation in a growing jaw usually is—and how this is imaged in a panoramic X-ray.

# 7 Evaluation of Space Conditions and Growth Changes

# 8 Abnormalities of Dentitional Development

# 9 Abnormalities of the Facial Skeleton and Soft Tissues

# Preface

The development of the human dentition is a continuous and extremely complex biological process. Moreover, it is normal for many variations in topogenesis and structure of the teeth and the jaws to occur over time. Pathologies of the teeth and of the hard and soft tissues, of either developmental or acquired origin, are frequently found. Many of them are clinical problems and require diagnosis, long-term supervision, and interceptive and/or corrective treatment during childhood.

In recent decades panoramic X-rays have proved a clinically powerful diagnostic procedure, particularly in orthodontics and pedodontics. Panoramic X-rays provide one complete overall view of the developmental status of a child's dentition and orofacial structure. This technique provides information not only on various morphological details, but also on the time related aspects of dental development. Frequently this is essential in the decision process, for long-term planning in the surveillance of the patient's dental development, in monitoring treatment progress, and in evaluating results.

The panoramic technique has been adopted by clinicians to provide a first, leading entry to more detailed diagnostic X-ray investigations, if they are indicated. However, clinical and teaching experience has shown that interpretation of panoramic X-rays is difficult. Spatial imaginative faculties are essential to arrive at correct interpretations.

The aim of this atlas is to facilitate the interpretation of panoramic X-rays of the developing dentition. To that purpose the book demonstrates the effects of various positions of the facial skull and dentition relative to the X-ray machine and also studies in detail normal anatomical structures and their normal variations. A sequential method to analyse panoramic X-rays is presented.

The various development phases of teeth and jaws are demonstrated in representative X-rays. Particular attention is given to the real three-dimensional topography of common variations to evaluate their effect on image *formation and interpretation.*

Reconstructions of the dentition were made from dry child skull preparations. Panoramic X-rays of these reconstructions, combined with photographs and drawings, effectively visualise the real complexity of the anatomy.

Abnormalities of the dentition and the jaws and orofacial tissues as seen in panoramic X-rays in clinical conditions are presented with representative examples. There is no attempt at completeness in this respect, but the most common abnormalities have been selected. Aspects of the analysis of space conditions in the mixed and adolescent dentition and evaluations of changes in serial panoramic X-rays are discussed. The various practical uses of the panoramic X-rays are all given attention.

This book is an atlas. The presentation of information is essentially visual, with the text limited to discussion of features necessary for effective understanding of the illustrations. It is designed in such a way that the reader becomes involved in the procedure of evaluating a child's developing dentition, and of making a diagnosis.

Where appropriate the X-rays are arranged without any signs or markers. Line drawings with markers printed in red and explanatory legends are placed so that the reader can cover up these drawings and train himself in interpreting images.

In a book like this the quality of reproduction of X-rays is crucial. All possible care has been taken to obtain and select the best pictures. However, in a few rare clinical situations the choice had to be made between deletion of that condition from the book or inclusion of a suboptimal X-ray. In almost all instances the original X-ray was used to produce the illustrations.

It is hoped that this information serves to increase knowledge and understanding of the development of the human dentition and orofacial structures and contributes to improved clinical performance.

May this book enhance the proper use of panoramic X-rays. Optimal interpretation will prevent unnecessary radiographs.

This book should be of particular interest to dentists, pedodontists, orthodontists, oral surgeons, anatomists, and dental and medical radiologists, as well as medical specialists in ear, nose, and throat medicine, plastic surgery, and students taking courses in development of dentition, clinical pedodontics, orthodontics, or oral diagnosis. It may also be of help in forensic and medico-legal cases.

Maastricht, Spring 1990.

# Acknowledgements

The author is indebted to the following persons:

Henk W.B. Jansen Ph.D., University of Groningen, who contributed to Chapter 4.

Prof. Dr. Frans P.G.M. van der Linden, University of Nijmegen, and Prof. Dr. Birthe Prahl-Andersen, University of Amsterdam, for many thought provoking discussions over the past 25 years.

Jef M.M. Crefcoeur, orthodontist, Maastricht, who made his vast collection of material available and inspired me in many ways.

Staff members of the Department of Orthodontics, University of Groningen; in particular: Bert Jongsma Ph.D., Maria Chàvez-Lomeli Ph.D., Arie van Zwol, Johan Perdok, and Marjolein Scheffer; and Marcella Kreuze, formerly at the University of Groningen Department of Orthodontics; all of whom helped in many ways.

Ruurd Koopmans and Hans Mays, oral surgeons at the Department of Oral Surgery, Academic Hospital, University of Limburg, Maastricht, who advised on the interpretation of several X-rays.

Tsjerk de Jager, orthodontist, Department of Orthodontics, University of Groningen, with whom I designed a teaching course on the development of dentition that formed the inspirational basis for this book.

Peter van Harteveld, who made many of the panoramic X-rays.

H. Flanderijn, who made the drawings for Chapters 3 and 6.

Lucia Lejeune, who prepared the manuscript.

Fridy Duterloo, who compiled the index.

8

# 1 Introduction

## 1.1 Introduction

The first part of this chapter briefly reviews historical aspects of the development of panoramic radiology. In the second part the current literature on the development of the human dentition is discussed, and some recommendations for literary study are made. Finally, the clinical indications for taking panoramic X-rays in children are discussed.

## 1.2 Panoramic Radiology

Panoramic radiology underwent a long developmental period before the technique became universally accepted for clinical use. Today the technique is recognised as an important advancement in modern dentistry.

As early as 1933 in Japan[61] and 1943 in Germany[36] the possibilities of making a one-film-one-shot projection of the complete dental arches were being investigated. In the fifties and sixties the bases for the current techniques were established with the fundamental research work of the Finnish scientist Yrjö V. Paatero[75]. After years of experimentation, he developed the orthopantomograph, producing a continuous image with adequate resolution of details. This machine has since been produced and improved by various manufacturers. A slightly different apparatus, working on the same basic principles but producing a split image (Panorex), was marketed in the United States after a design by J. W. Kumpala and D. C. Hudson[34].

In the late sixties and seventies panoramic X-ray machines came into widespread clinical use.

Then, rapidly, the diagnostic possibilities, the advantages and disadvantages, became the subject of many publications. A number of books on the technique itself were published [6,42,49].

Soon the advantages for routine evaluation of the developmental status of the dentition became obvious. Particularly for orthodontic and pedodontic patients, the panoramic X-ray provided an unprecedented means of obtaining a complete overview of the developing dentition.

The panoramic technique replaced the tedious and often difficult procedure of taking a series of fragmentary individual dental films. With dental films, it is often difficult to obtain satisfactory exposures in children, and retakes often need to be made. The panoramic technique usually provides a sufficiently reliable overview, so that other, detailed, X-rays are only needed in complicated and exceptional cases and localised areas.

Moreover, in general the radiation dose is less than when a series of dental films is made.

The greatest disadvantage of the technique, as it is today, is the impossibility of standardisation. Standardisation of observation or measurement technique is the basis for adequate growth studies. For research purposes, this shortcoming of the panoramic technique is very serious. It is beyond the scope of this introduction to describe the causes; suffice it to say that it is in part the inherent characteristics of the technique, and in part the complicated process of growth and development of the dentition and the dentofacial complex, that make accurate longitudinal studies impossible. For clinical evaluations, however, some possibilities do exist.

Valuable large-scale cross-sectional studies of growth and development of the dentition with the use of panoramic X-rays were made: for instance, on the prevalence of hypo- and hyperodontia[1,28], on tooth formation age[30], and on aspects of eruption[9].

# 1.3 Development of the Dentition

To understand the contents of this atlas, previous knowledge of the development of the dentition is helpful, but not necessary. However, for the clinical management of problems of a child's dentition, additional knowledge is essential.

Information selected with that purpose includes histological development, topographical anatomy of the developing dentition, arch form changes, occlusal developmental changes, genetics, and numerical data for clinical reference. As a field it is too large to be covered in this atlas.

The reader is recommended to consult the following works.

Histological development of the teeth and other oral structures is very well described in A. R. Ten Cate, *Oral histology: development, structure and function*[76]. Tadahiro Ooë (*Human tooth and dental arch development*) describes and demonstrates in fine drawings of reconstructions the early relative positions of tooth germs[62].

Topographical illustrations of dentitional development in dry skull preparations are shown in F.P.G.M. van der Linden and H.S. Duterloo, *Development of the human dentition —an atlas*[78].

Arch form changes and occlusal development have been described in a longitudinal study by R.E. Moyers, F.P.G.M. van der Linden, M.L. Riolo, and J.A. McNamara Jr, *Standards of human occlusal development*[59].

A review of genetics of dental development has been presented by S.M. Garn in: *Biology of occlusal development*[24]. This volume also contains other valuable studies on dentitional development.

A valuable recent introductory overview on the subject has been published by F.P.G.M. van der Linden, *Development of the dentition*[80].

A series of studies of great clinical value have been published by C.F.A. Moorrees[53-7]. Further, several orthodontic textbooks contain informative chapters on dentitional development and clinical management of developmental problems[26,58,77].

# 1.4 Clinical Indications for Taking Panoramic X-rays in Children

The decision to make a panoramic X-ray of the dentition of a child can only be made responsibly after anamnesis and thorough intraoral examination.

This intraoral examination should include at least digital palpation of the buccal and lingual mucosa and the retromolar areas (the presence of many unerupted teeth can be palpated); a judgement of mucosa, occlusions and general conditions should be made; the teeth should be counted, identified (deciduous or permanent), checked for mobility, and compared with the age of the child.

Then, after completion of the intraoral examination, it is good practice first to consider carefully whether a panoramic X-ray is actually indicated in this case, and, if so, whether the right moment to make it has arrived, and what one actually will do with the expected information.

In general one should wait until the age of approximately 7 or 8 years for a panoramic X-ray. That is the time of the end of the first transitional stage, when the permanent incisors have emerged. The reason for this is that the developmental stage of the dentition makes these lower ages less than optimal. The presence of several permanent teeth may be undetectable. In addition, when, for instance, hypodontia or hyperodontia is found, active measures intended to do something about the problem usually have to wait until further development. That renders the panoramic X-ray obsolete. Another common situation is the rising concern about the size and position of newly emerging permanent incisors and the diastemata that normally occur. It is better to follow the process of tooth emergence in such a situation and to wait for a panoramic X-ray until the first transition is completed, if no other urgent reason exists. By that time there may no longer be reason for concern.

In general one can say that a panoramic X-ray should confirm expectations derived from the intraoral examination, and that the X-ray should be taken at a moment as close as possible to the time one actually expects treat-ment to begin. Of course, there are exceptions to this rule; but it is, we must emphasise, good practice carefully to consider whether the right moment has arrived.

Obviously, many good reasons can be enumerated for taking a panoramic X-ray of a child, and if one such reason applies, one should proceed.

The view presented here will be repeated in several other places in this book. Insight into the normal development of the dentition and commonly occurring variations is necessary for correct judgements and appropriate action.

# 2 Working with the Panoramic X-ray Machine

## 2.1 Introduction

This chapter describes the methods, techniques, procedures, and materials used to produce the illustrations in the subsequent chapters. The X-ray machines, the craniostat, skeletal material, reconstructive procedures, and marking techniques are introduced. The effects of patient positioning are extensively discussed.

A dry child skull with a mixed dentition in the intertransitional stage is used as a standard model. Artefacts and technical errors are indicated.

## 2.2 Rotational Panoramic Radiography

In this section the essential elements will be given of the theory of this very specific projection technique. For an in-depth overview of the field the reader should consult Welander *et al.*, 1982[83].

In panoramic radiography the X-ray source is provided with a narrow slit vertical diaphragm that produces a slit beam. The X-ray source rotates around the object (the patient's head).

The cassette with the film is attached to the rotating system and moves in the same direction as the beam. The film is given a correct speed by opposing this movement with a contrary movement relative to the beam, so that during rotation a different part of the film is continuously exposed.

The rotation centre of the beam is the functional focus of the projection. The movements of the film and the X-ray source affect the length of the image recorded on the film in the horizontal plane. In the vertical plane the height enlargement in the image remains the same as long as the distances between the X-ray source and the object and between the object and the film remain the same.

The result is a sharply depicted object plane. Either toward the rotation centre of the beam or toward the film, objects have a different speed, resulting in increased blurring in both directions from that plane.

In this way a zone in the patient's head is imaged with sufficient resolution that objects in this zone can be distinguished. This zone is called the image layer.

The position of the image layer is dependent on the film speed. Increase of the speed of film moves the image layer away from the rotation centre; a decrease moves the layer closer to the rotation centre. This also influences the layer thickness. With acceleration and deceleration, the position and the thickness of the image layer relative to the film and the rotation centre of the beam can thus be manipulated.

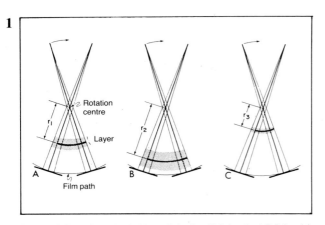

Fig. 1. The position of the layer is dependent on the speed of the film. Increase of the speed of film moves the image layer away from the rotation centre; a decrease moves the layer closer to the rotation centre. This also influences the layer thickness. With acceleration and deceleration the position and the thickness of the image layer relative to the film and the rotation centre of the beam can thus be manipulated. A = constant speed. B = constant increased speed. C = constant decreased speed. Speed acceleration and deceleration, changing from A to B and B to C, changes the position and thickness of the image layer.

Figures 1, 2, 3, 4 and 6 reprinted with permission from O.E. Langland, R.P. Langlais, and C.R. Morris, *Principles and practice of panoramic radiology*. Malvern, Pennsylvania: Lea & Febiger, 1982.

## 2.2.1 Projection of the Dental Arches and the Jaws

The dental arches and the jaws are not circular or elliptic. Adaptations are thus necessary to fit the image layer as perfectly as possible to the average jaw. Manufacturers of panoramic X-ray machines have done this by experimenting with rotation centres and film speed.

The simplest method is a projection with one stationary rotation centre (for example,

the S.S. White Panorex). The rotation centre is in a fixed position and the patient is moved in a second position, giving a split image. Other machines have three fixed rotation centres, or a combination of stationary and moving or continuously sliding rotation centres. These techniques create a continuous image.

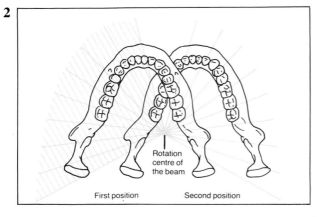

Fig. 2. The machine has one fixed rotation centre in the beam; two effective centres are created by moving the patient. The X-ray is taken in two sequences, and a split image results.

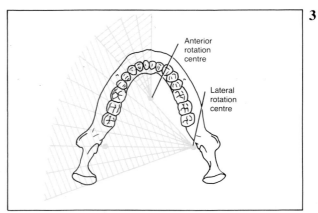

Fig. 3. Three fixed rotation centres are used, leading to a continuous image (Siemens OP1).

Fig. 4. A continuously sliding rotation centre is used in the Siemens OP5.

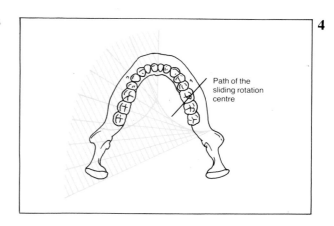

Path of the sliding rotation centre

## 2.2.2 The Image Layer and Aspects of Enlargement, Reduction and Distortion

The shape of the dental arches and the position of (unerupted) teeth vary considerably among individuals. Particularly in cases with developing dentitions and in cases with malocclusions and ectopically positioned teeth, there are always compromises to be taken into account. Problems of fit of the standard image layer exist in almost all situations. Some blurring and dullness, variable enlargement and distortion unavoidably occur and must be dealt with. It is important to know within what limits the panoramic X-ray is reliable enough for diagnostic purposes.

Fig. 5. Image layer characteristics. The shape of the image layer of the Siemens OP2 has been used for this illustration.

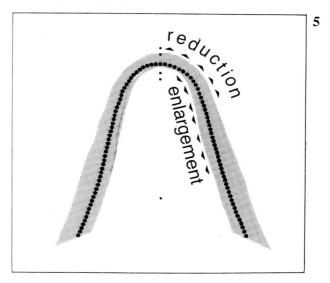

reduction

enlargement

The image layer has roughly the shape of the dental arch. The plane of the highest degree of sharpness (stipple line) is in the middle of the layer. Objects within the shaded area are imaged with acceptable resolution. Objects more buccal or lingual are increasingly blurred. The rotation centre of the beam, which is the functional focus of projection, is positioned lingually to the image layer. Therefore objects positioned more lingually are enlarged more than objects positioned toward the buccal. Long straight objects (like an incisor) that are positioned at one end buccally and at the other end lingually to the plane of greatest clarity may thus be seen as curved.

Moreover, in going from mesial to distal there is a gradually *increasing* linear enlargement factor.

15

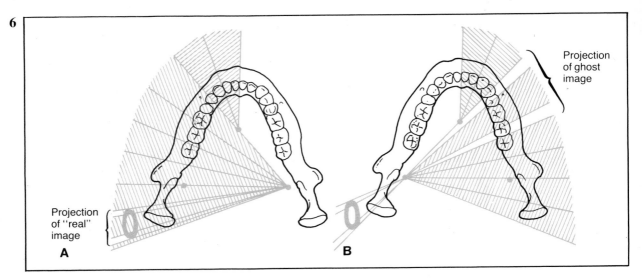

Fig. 6. Ghost images.

Ghost images are the result of the projection of objects that are positioned between the X-ray source and the centre of rotation of the beam. As they are outside the image layer, they are vaguely blurred, seen at the side of the film opposite to where they are in reality. The above diagram illustrates how a ghost image of an earring is projected. Such an image is seen in Figs. 372/373, page 214. See also the remarks in section 2.6, page 31.

## 2.3 The Craniostat

To produce special panoramic X-rays for this atlas and other research purposes, a craniostat was built (see Figs. 7/8).

This craniostat fits exactly into the plexiglass dome of the orthopantomograph (Siemens OP2) and can easily be installed in the standard position and removed. Dry skulls can repeatedly be placed in various exactly reproducible positions.

The occlusal plane was kept horizontal, with an accurately fitting acrylic bite fork. Elastic bands are used to keep the mandible in position.

The construction of this craniostat made it possible to work out various experimental conditions without interference with the normal clinical work.

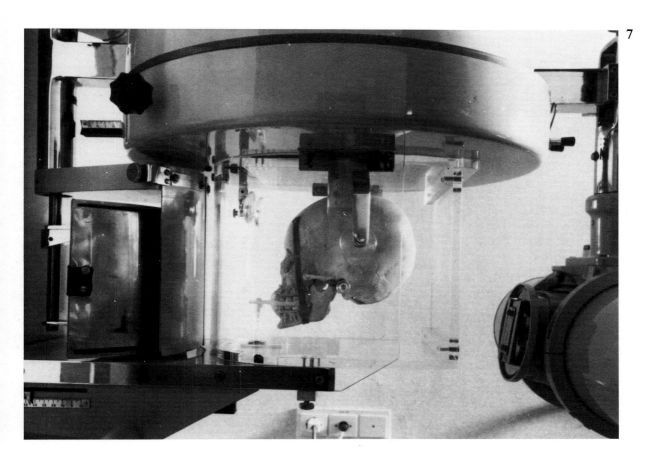

Fig. 7. Orthopantomograph with craniostat and dry skull in position.

Fig. 8. Craniostat with dry skull.

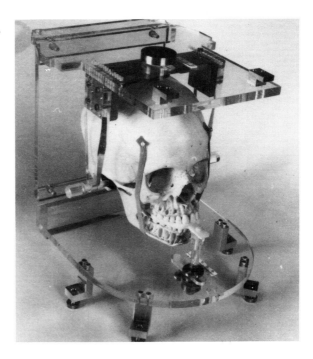

# 2.3.1 Selection of Dry Skeletal Material

**9**

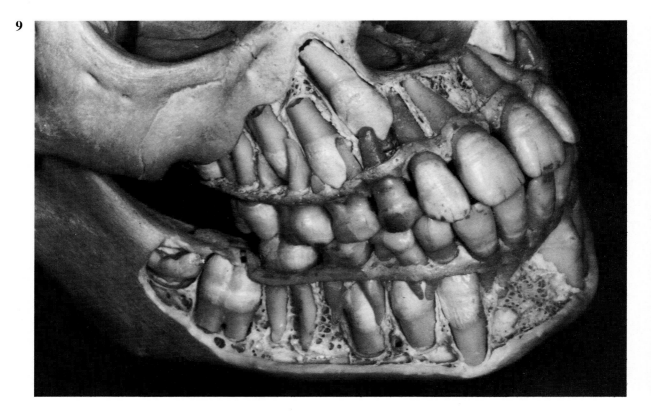

Fig. 9. Photograph detail: dentition from right.

A well preserved complete child skull (approximately 9 years of age) was selected. The dentition is in the intertransitional stage. The dental arches are complete and well formed. The buccal cortex was pared away to expose the unerupted teeth and the roots of the erupted teeth. Figs. 9–12 show the dry skull preparation, intertransitional stage.

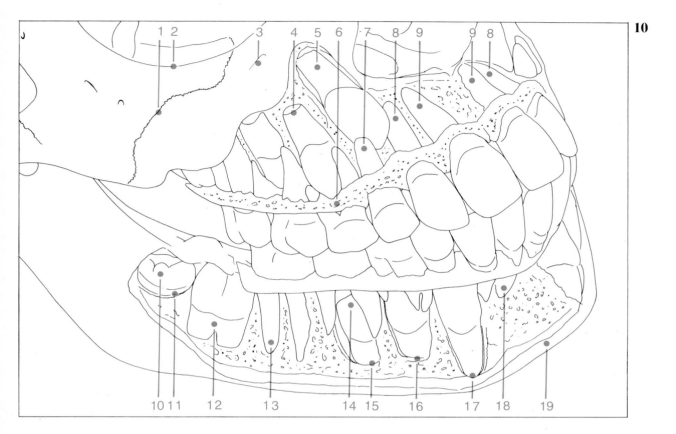

Fig. 10. Drawing of Fig. 9. 1. Sutura zygomaticomaxillaris. 2. Inferior border of the orbita. 3. Foramen infraorbitale. 4. Forming root of permanent maxillary first premolar. Its crown is between the roots of the deciduous first molar. 5. Forming root of permanent maxillary canine. Note the high position of the unerupted canine directly lateral to the apertura piriformis. The tip of its crown is lingual to the root end of the deciduous canine; its mesial edge buccal to the root of the permanent lateral incisor. 6. The bifurcation of the deciduous first molar is uncovered, indicating bone resorption at the alveolar crest. 7. Root of deciduous maxillary canine. Note the amount of root not covered by bone below the alveolar crest. 8. Permanent lateral incisors. 9. Permanent central incisors. The forming apices of the incisors are still close to the floor of the nose. 10. Permanent mandibular third molar crown partly formed in its crypt. 11. The fundus of the crypt is a smooth, thin, cortical plate. 12. The roots of the unerupted permanent mandibular second molar are forming. The root bifurcation has just been established. 13. The apices of the permanent mandibular first molar are nearly complete. 14. The crown of the permanent second premolar is located between the roots of the deciduous second molar. 15. Fundus of the crypt of the second premolar. 16. Fundus of the crypt of the first premolar. The fundus of both crypts is a smooth, thin, cortical layer. 17. The formative area of the root of the unerupted mandibular permanent canine is buccally positioned at the mandibular cortex. 18. The roots of the erupted mandibular incisors are more lingually positioned, and these teeth procline. 19. The cortex of the symphysis.

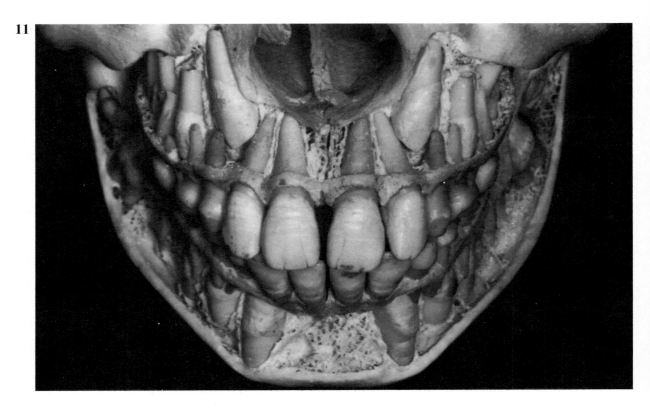

Fig. 11. Frontal view from above.

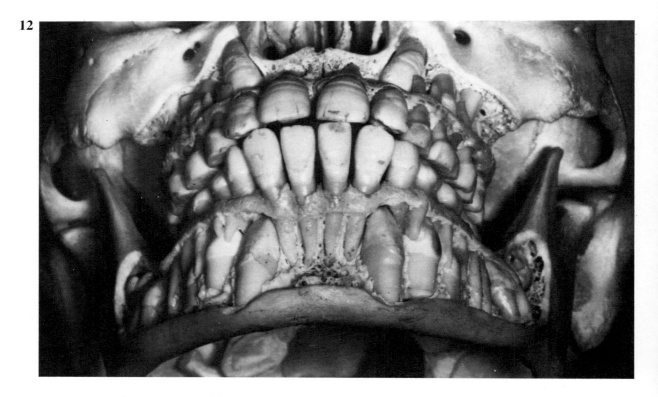

Fig. 12. Frontal view from below.

# 2.3.2 Standard Panoramic X-ray

With the help of the craniostat a series of panoramic X-rays was made in various symmetrical positions. One position was marked as the standard reference. The image layer is then in optimal position with the least distortion and differences in enlargement between the teeth (Figs. 13–15).

The standard panoramic X-ray is used as a reference for evaluation of effects of variations in position of the skull dealt with in the following section.

The standard reference position was also used for the detailed anatomical studies with lead reference markers that are dealt with in Chapter 3.

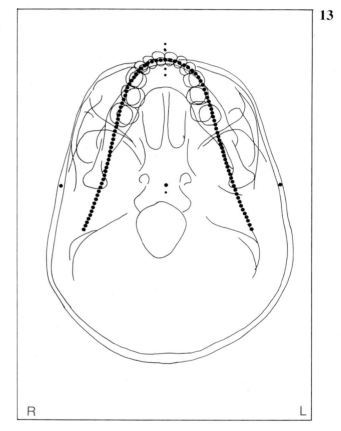

Fig. 13. Tracing of basilar cephalogram of skull. The position of the image layer for the standard panoramic X-ray is optimal.

**14**

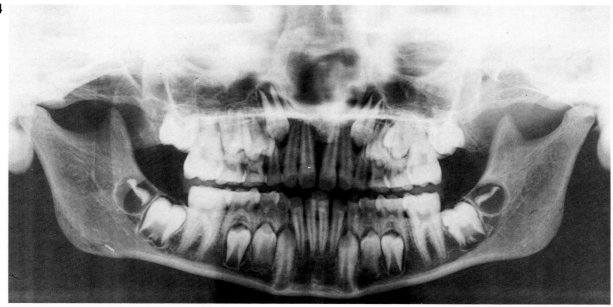

Fig. 14. Panoramic X-ray of the dry skull preparation of Figs. 9–12 taken in standard reference position˙.

**15**

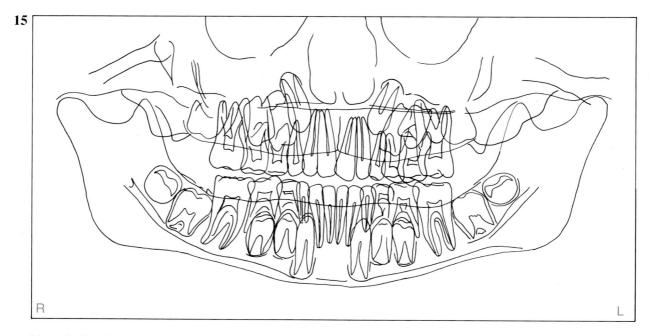

R                                                                                                                    L

Fig. 15. Tracing of standard panoramic X-ray. Note the horizontal projection of the occlusal plane and the image of the acrylic splint.

˙ All panoramic X-rays, either complete or as a detail, are shown as if the reader is looking from the outside of the mouth towards the oral cavity, the left side of the patient's face being to the reader's right. R thus indicates the patient's right side, L the left side.

# 2.3.3  Effects of Positional Variation

Positional variations were analysed in three ways:

1.  Horizontal backward–forward positions.

2.  Rotation around a horizontal transversal axis through the right and left porions.
3.  Rotation around a vertical axis at 90° angles to the horizontal transversal axis.

## 2.3.3.1  *Horizontal backward–forward positions.*

Fig. 16. The position of the image layer is too far backward; the skull is too far forward.

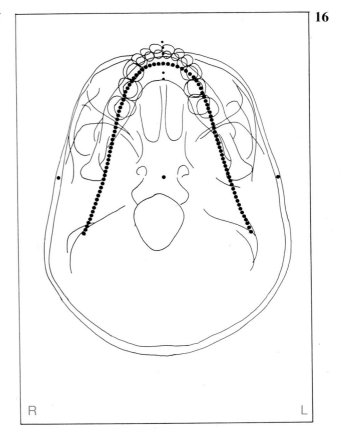

**16**

R                    L

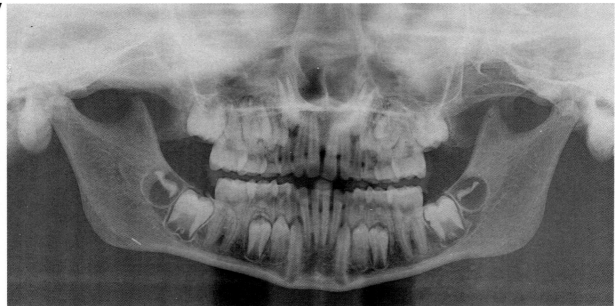

Fig. 17. Panoramic X-ray: skull too far forward.

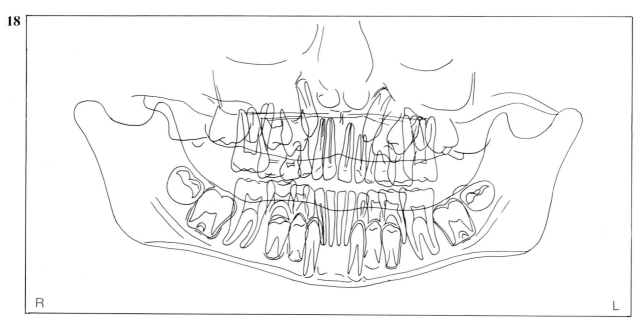

Fig. 18. Drawing of Fig. 17. The frontal teeth are imaged too narrowly, and there is increased overlap of teeth in the buccal regions. Note that the total width of the image is also decreased in the horizontal dimension. The cusps of deciduous molars and permanent first molars appear too large; this is due to their lingual position relative to the image layer.

Fig. 19. The position of the image layer is too far forward; the skull, too far backward.

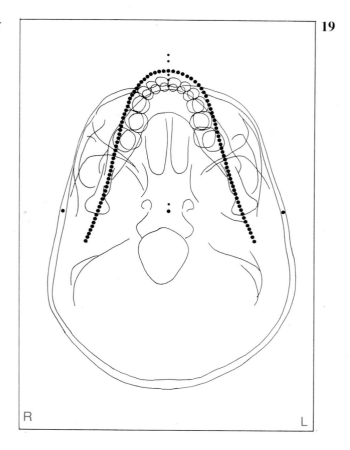

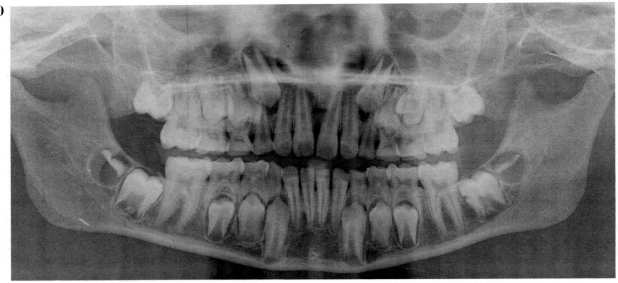

**20**

Fig. 20. Panoramic X-ray: skull too far backward.

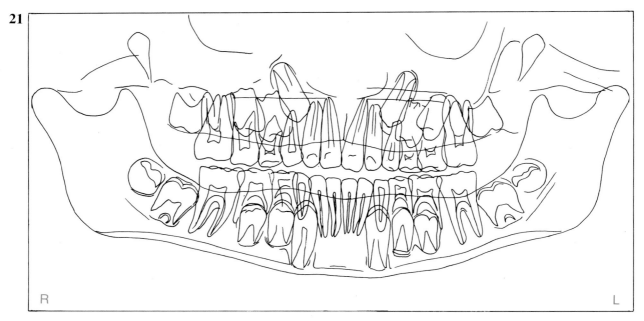

**21**

R                                                                                    L

Fig. 21. Drawing of Fig. 20. The frontal teeth are imaged too broadly; the total image of the jaws is greatly increased in the horizontal dimension.

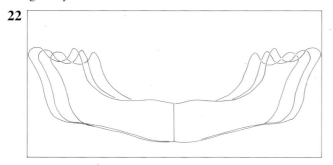

**22**

Fig. 22. Superposition of the outlines of the mandibles of the X-rays of "too far forward", "standard", and "too far backward" positions.

## 2.3.3.2 *Rotation around a horizontal transversal axis.*

Two panoramic X-rays are shown: 10° frontal upward and 10° frontal downward rotation.

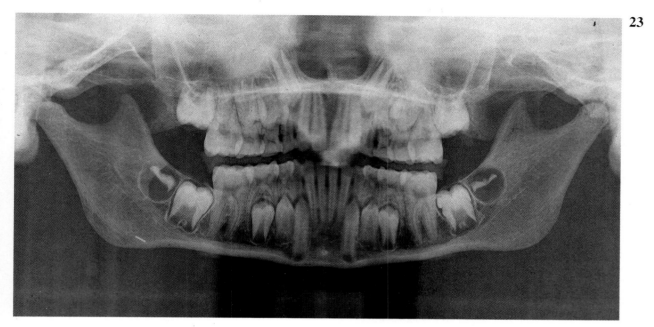

Fig. 23. Panoramic X-ray: 10° front up.

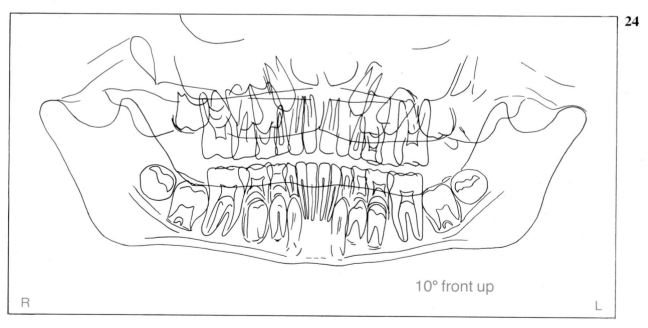

Fig. 24. Drawing of Fig. 23. The results of this rotation are a decreased horizontal dimension in the frontal region, and blurring. Note also the appearance of diastemata as the teeth reach optimum resolution. The occlusal plane is inverted with the front up.

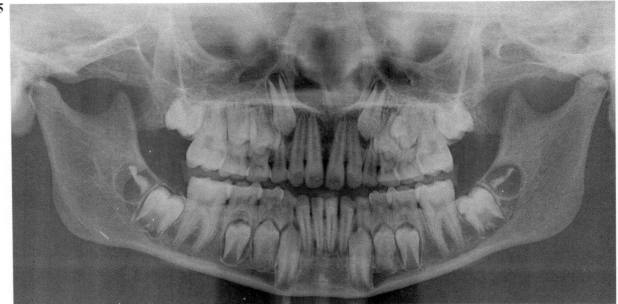

Fig. 25. Panoramic X-ray: 10° front down.

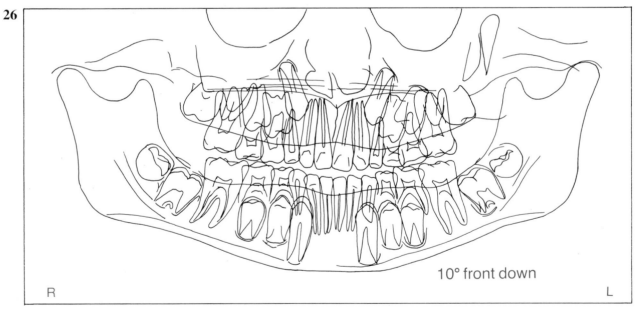

Fig. 26. Drawing of Fig. 25. This image is of rather good quality. The occlusal plane is slightly curved. Compare the shape of the mandible to that in Figs. 23/24. Manufacturers frequently advise this position for patients, because the externally visible plane porion/subnasale (Campers' plane) is then approximately horizontal, and the image is usually good.

## 2.3.3.3 *Rotation around a central vertical axis.*

Fig. 27. Position of the image layer. The skull is rotated 10° to the left around a central vertical axis.

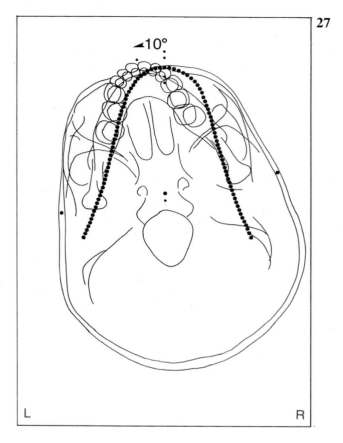

**28**

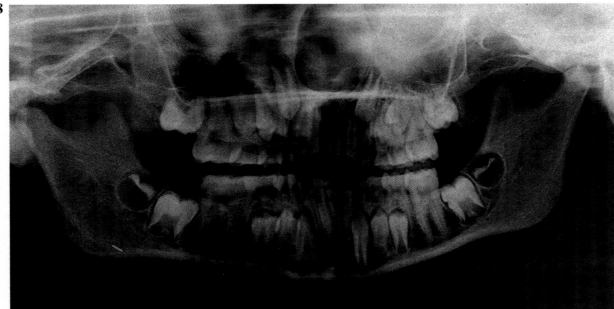

Fig. 28. Panoramic X-ray: 10° toward left.

**29**

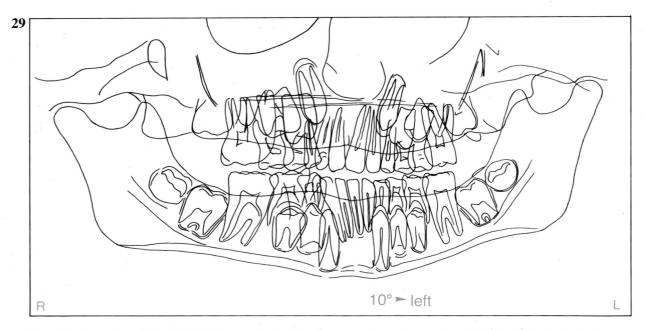

Fig. 29. Drawing of Fig. 28. 10° toward left. The front teeth incline to the right side. The left side buccal teeth are imaged too narrowly, while at the right side the buccal teeth are too wide. Note also the asymmetry of the mandible.

30

## 2.4  Reconstructive Procedures

The buccal alveolar cortex was removed with fine dental burs. The teeth were pared free and removed from their sockets and crypts. The acrylic splint was used as a base structure to make reconstructions and other setups of the teeth without the skull. The reconstructions were X-rayed in standard position. These panoramic X-rays are discussed in Chapter 6.

## 2.5  Marking Techniques

Soft lead wire (diameter 0.5 mm) and metallic balls (diameter 0.7 mm) were used as markers for anatomical structures to be identified on the standard panoramic X-ray.

Implants were placed at both sides of sutures at several locations in the maxilla, particularly in the sphenopterygoid fissure, the nasal apertura, and the zygomata. Each time only a few markers were placed, the X-ray taken, and the procedure then repeated with other markers. In this way confusing images were avoided.

## 2.6  Handling Films

All films, clinical as well as experimental, were processed with standardised automatic developing machines, according to the instructions of the manufacturers.

## 2.7  Common Artefacts

When a panoramic X-ray is first interpreted one should check for symmetry and image quality of the teeth. The previous paragraphs showed that patient position is of utmost importance. Distinction should be made between abnormal asymmetry of the patient and asymmetrical positioning of the normal patient.

Ghost images are seen when earrings, etc., are worn by the patient during taking of the X-ray. They may obscure areas of interest and should be avoided. See Figs. 372/373, page 214.

Ghost images of the hardpalate are frequently seen (see Figs. 104/105, point 7, pages 88–89), usually overlapping the maxillary sinus of the opposite site. Many of the undefined, indistinct shadows seen in this area are ghost images of nasal structures or even of the mandibular ramus and condyle on the other side.

Other rather frequently seen artefacts are caused by movements of the child during the rotation of the machine. Such movement artefacts can be very misleading; in other cases the artefact is obvious. Not in all situations is a retake necessary.

When X-raying children, special care should be taken to create an atmosphere of trust and tranquillity. Explain clearly to the child what happens. Panoramic X-rays, to evaluate dentitional development, should preferably not be taken before the age of 7 or 8.

Only in exceptional circumstances should panoramic X-rays of young children be made. Before 7 years of age the chance that late developing teeth will not be seen is relatively large, and in general not very much can be done about such conditions at that young age.

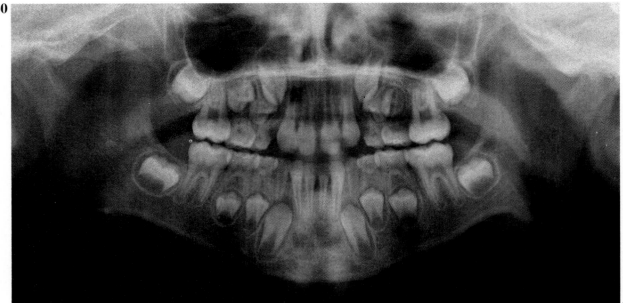

Fig. 30.  Panoramic X-ray: boy 8.1 years old.

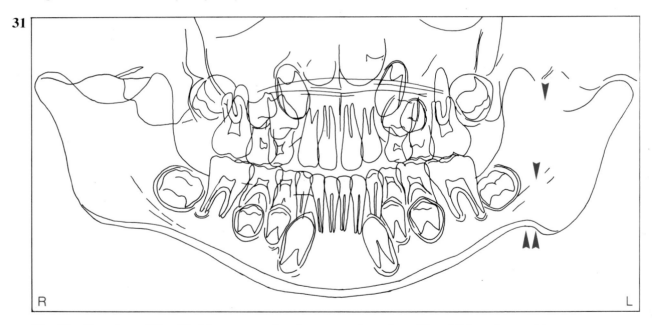

Fig. 31.  Drawing of Fig. 30. Movement of patient caused artefact. The child made a sudden movement at the beginning of the rotation of the machine. The image is particularly misleading, as such a morphology of the mandibular ramus, with marked antegonial notching (arrows), appears also in relation to condylar growth disturbances. See section 9.4, pages 213–219.

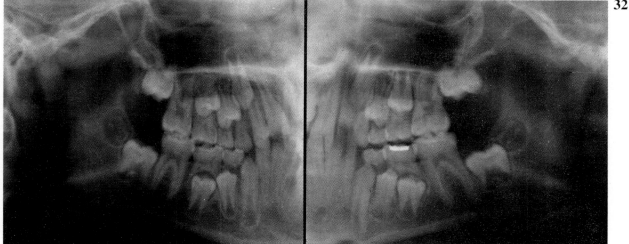

Fig. 32. Panoramic X-ray: boy 11.2 years old.

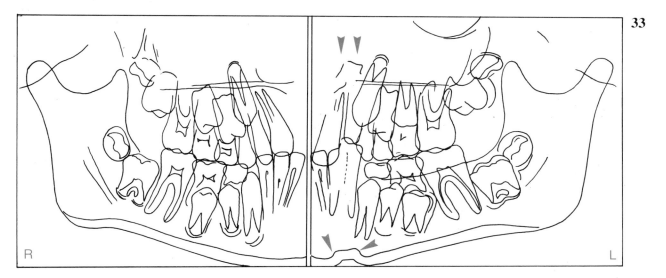

Fig. 33. Drawing of Fig. 32. Sudden vertical movement during rotational movement of the machine. Note the sharp disruption of the mandibular cortex and the blurred image of the lateral incisor region in the left mandible and maxilla (arrows).

# 3 Normal Anatomy of the Facial Region and Dentition

## 3.1 Introduction

The head and neck constitute one of the most complicated regions of the human body. Thorough knowledge of this region—not only of the morphology of the bones of the skull and vertebrae, but also detailed insight into internal structures and their relative position— is essential for the correct interpretation of panoramic X-rays.

Careful study of an atlas of normal anatomy (for example, *Color atlas of head and neck anatomy,* by R.M.H. McMinn, R.T. Hutchings, and B. Logan, Chicago: Year Book Medical Publishers, 1981) is strongly recommended, as this forms the basis for good clinical diagnosis[52].

In panoramic X-rays the complex structures of the facial skull and dentition are imaged distorted and variably enlarged. The clinician, therefore, is confronted at once with a large number of various structures. Teaching experience has shown that it is an excess of information presented simultaneously that, in addition to the factors mentioned before, leads to errors of interpretation and/or overlooked diagnoses.

In this chapter a sequential procedure is presented to help to analyse a panoramic X-ray. Then a standard X-ray of a dry skull preparation is analysed in great detail. These illustrations can also be used as a reference.

Normally, in clinical situations some of the structures seen in these illustrations are not, or only vaguely or partly seen, for a variety of reasons.

It should be mentioned here that a panoramic X-ray is taken primarily to image the dentition. Other facial structures are seen, but the X-ray is not taken specifically to study these structures. There are special X-ray techniques to study skull structures, but their description is extraneous to the theme of this atlas.

The nomenclature used in this atlas is, as far as possible, the one used by McMinn, Hutchings, and Logan[52].

## 3.1.1 Systematic Analysis of Panoramic X-rays

Use a light box that is framed to the rim of the film; use a magnifying glass to see details if necessary.

It is important first to make a general survey:

1. Is there proper exposure, light and dark areas, contrast?

2. What is the position of the image relative to the borders of the film?
3. Is it symmetrical? If not, why? What about patient position?
4. Are there obvious artefacts, technical errors, or blurred areas that prevent proper interpretation?

## 3.1.2 The Five Topographical Regions

The panoramic X-ray is divided into five topographical anatomical regions. Each of the regions is sequentially studied. Because the panoramic X-ray is bilateral, it is always possible to compare right and left sides. In this way information can be ordered and effectively noted.

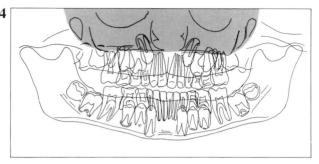

Fig. 34. The nasomaxillary region. This region comprises the zygomas, maxillary sinus, nasal septum, nasal conchae, apertura piriformis, hard palate, soft palate, and anterior nasal spine. It is the upper medial part of the X-ray.

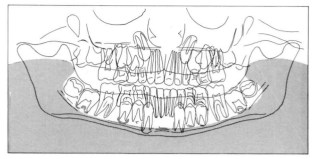

Fig. 35. The mandibular region comprises the body and ramus of the mandible and the soft tissues surrounding it: mandibular contour, symphysis, mental foramina, mandibular canal, mandibular angle, antegonial notch, tongue, pharynx, epiglottis, and hyoid bone. It constitutes the lower central and lateral parts of the X-ray.

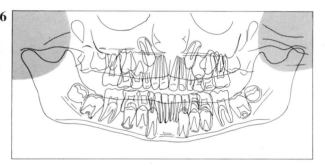

Fig. 36. The temporomandibular joint regions, mandibular condyle, temporal fossa, coronoid process, pterygoid regions, and maxillary tuberosity. It constitutes the upper lateral parts of the X-ray.

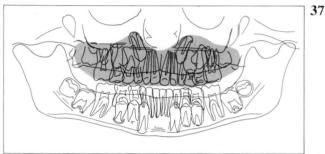

Fig. 37. Maxillary dentition. Noted are: number, identity, position, and formation stage of all teeth. Alveolar structures, dental crypts, root resorption deciduous teeth. Start at the right side.

Particularly in cases with a developing dentition with deciduous and permanent teeth present, it is important to count the teeth and identify them.

Other records, such as dental casts, cephalograms, and other X-rays can also be used to arrive at an integrated diagnosis of the case. Sometimes confirmation of an observation is necessary, and extra X-rays need to be taken for a special purpose. This can be decided after study of the panoramic X-ray.

Each of the five regions is now presented in detail, using the dry skull of a child of approximately 9 years.

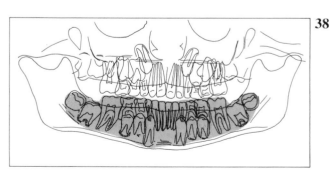

Fig. 38. Mandibular dentition. Noted are: number, identity, position, and formation stage of all teeth. Alveolar structures, dental crypts, root resorption deciduous teeth. Start at the left side.

## 3.2 The Nasomaxillary Region

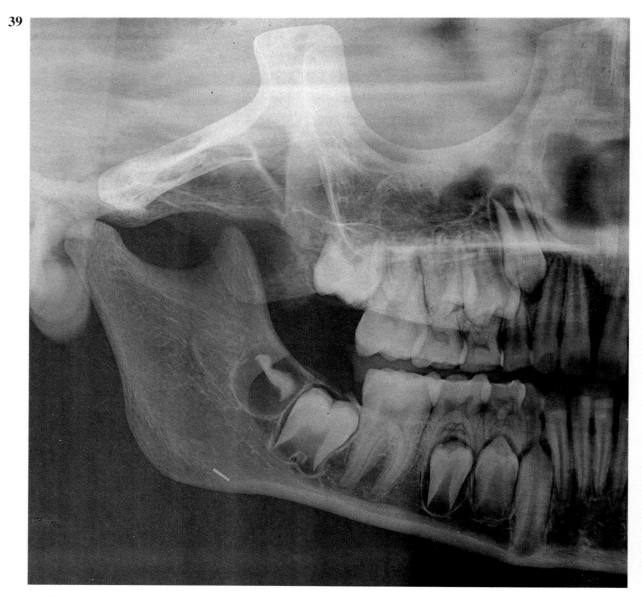

Fig. 39. Right half of panoramic X-ray of dry skull in standard position. Nasomaxillary region.

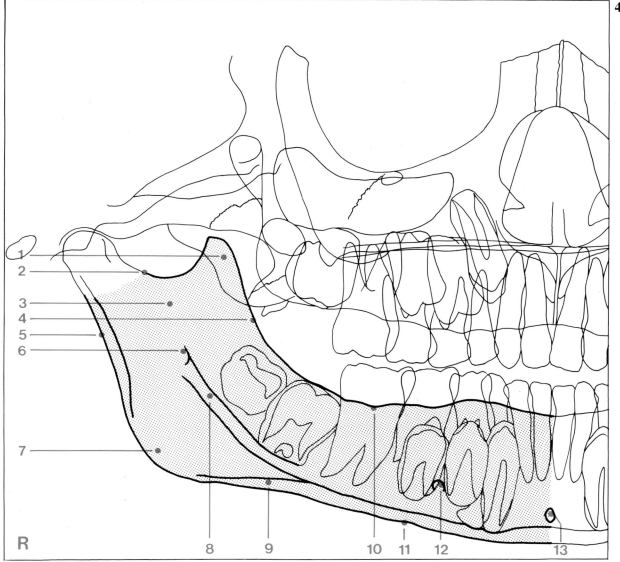

Fig. 42. Drawing of Fig. 41. The mandibular region. 1. Coronoid process. 2. Mandibular notch. 3. Mandibular ramus. 4. Anterior border of ramus. 5. Posterior border of ramus; cortex. 6. Mandibular foramen and lingula. 7. Mandibular angle. 8. Mandibular canal. 9. Antegonial notch. 10. Alveolar crest. 11. Lower border of mandible; mandibular cortex. 12. Mental foramen. The removal of the buccal cortical plate has influenced the image of the foramen. It is often, but not always, seen in X-rays. See also Figs. 360/361, page 209. 13. Mental spines.

# 3.3.1 Variations in Position and Shape of the Mandible

Contrasting shapes of the facial skeleton give very different images in panoramic X-rays.

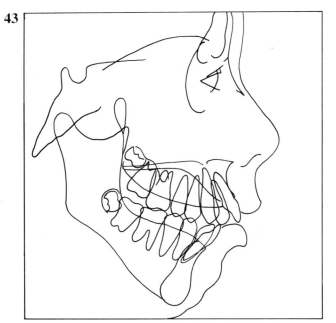

Fig. 43. A vertically overdeveloped convex face, often combined with Angle Class II, Division 1 malocclusion. Note the large gonial angle and steep mandibular plane.

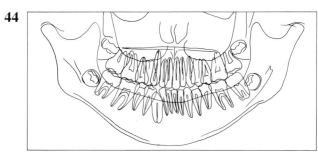

Fig. 44. Tracing of panoramic X-ray of the case of Fig. 43. Careful attention should be directed to head position relative to the X-ray machine in such cases. It might be necessary to keep Campers' plane slightly up in the frontal.

Fig. 45. Vertically underdeveloped concave face. Note the horizontal mandibular plane, small gonial angle and deep bite (Class II, Division 2). It may be advisable to have the patient bite on a cotton roll during exposure to avoid disturbing overprojections of teeth.

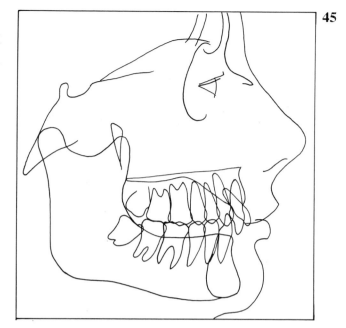

Fig. 46. Tracing of the panoramic X-ray of the case of Fig. 45. Compare Fig. 43 and Fig. 44 with Fig. 45 and Fig. 46 and note the constrasting morphology and resulting panoramic X-rays.

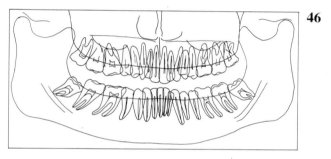

# 3.4 The Temporomandibular Joint Region

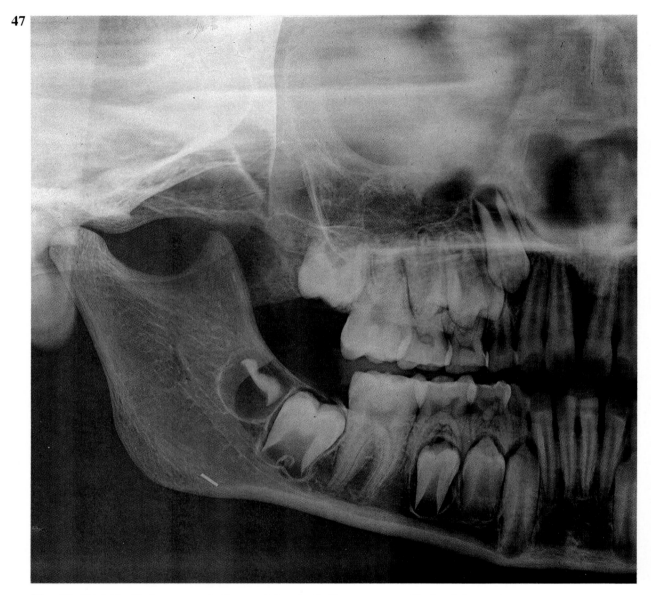

Fig. 47. Right half of panoramic X-ray of dry skull. Temporomandibular joint region.

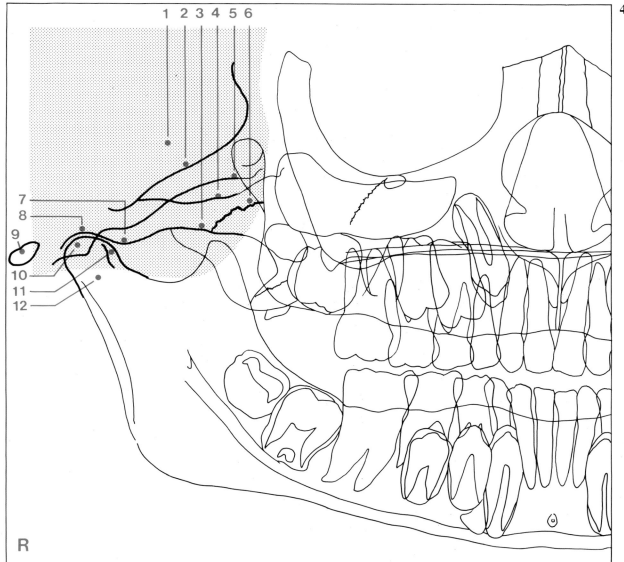

Fig. 48. Drawing of Fig. 47. The temporomandibular joint region. 1. Fossa cranii media. 2. Ala magna ossis sphenoidalis (endocranial cortex). 3. Margo inferior arcus zygomaticus. 4. Margo superior arcus zygomaticus. 5. Crista infratemporalis ossis sphenoidalis (ala magna). 6. Sutura zygomaticotemporalis. 7. Tuberculum articulare. 8. Fossa articularis (mandibular fossa). 9. External acoustic meatus. 10. Condylar process of mandible. 11. Pterygoid fovea. 12. Condylar neck.

## 3.4.1 The Shape of the Condyle

The shape of the condyle is of the utmost clinical importance, as the mandibular condyle forms a key growth region in the face.

In young children the condyles show as round structures, as in Figs. 47/48. Relatively frequently abnormal shapes are seen in aberrant facial growth patterns (see Section 9.4, pages 213 through 223).

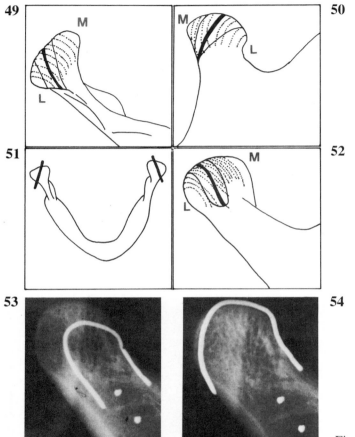

Figs. 49–54. Image formation of condylar surface.

Figs. 49–54 demonstrate which part of the condylar surface forms the image seen in an orthopantomogram. This was analysed by placing a successive series of lead wires over the surface of the condyles of 20 dry mandibles. It also shows (Figs. 53/54) that structures seen "inside" the condylar image may or may not be at the surface. This is something that cannot be determined[72]. The image of the condyle changes clearly with rotation of the head around a vertical axis, and very little with rotation around a horizontal axis, when a panoramic X-ray is taken.

It is important to state here that the panoramic X-rays are taken to study the dentition and are *not* made for the purpose of analysis of the condyle. If indicated, abnormal shapes observed in the panoramic X-ray might, however, lead to other special X-ray studies of the temporomandibular joints. This is a subject beyond the scope of this atlas.

Standard panoramic X-rays of the dentition are not suitable for analysis of dysfunctions of the temporomandibular joints, or for evaluation of condyle/fossa relationships.

# 3.5 The Maxillary Dentition Region

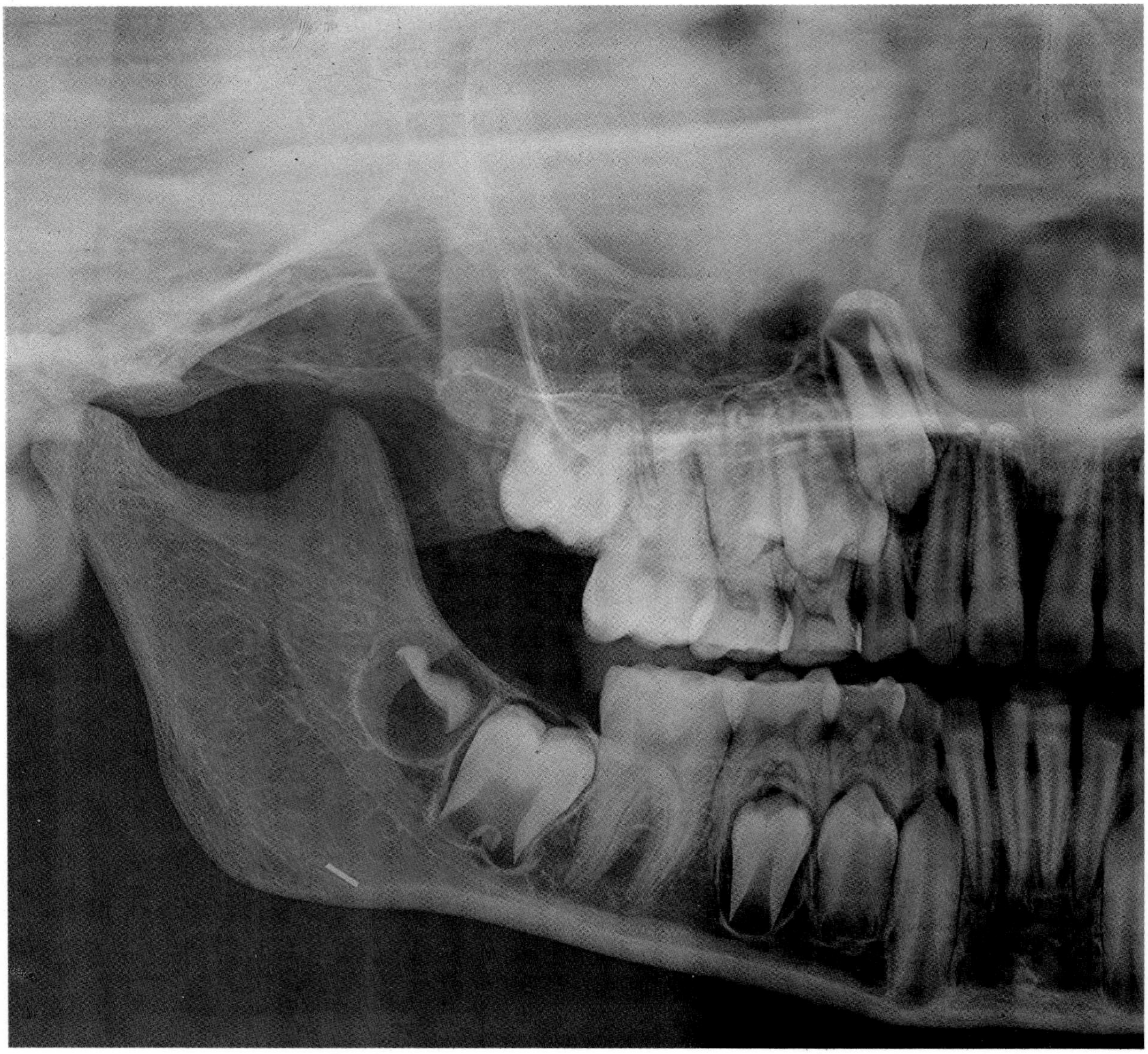

Fig. 55. Right half of panoramic X-ray of dry skull. Maxillary dentition.

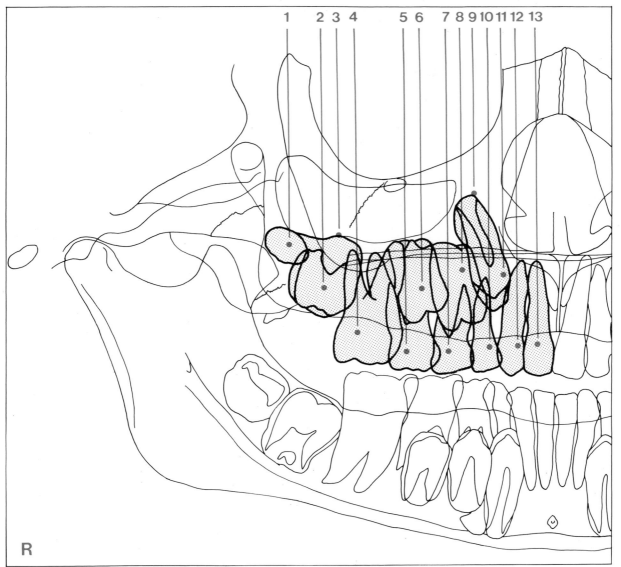

Fig. 56. Drawing of Fig. 55. The maxillary dentition. 1. Crypt of third molar. The crypt of the maxillary third molar is dorsally facing and wide open. In a dry skull preparation the developing crown is usually lost. 2. Maxillary second permanent molar. 3. Fundus of second and third molar crypts. The fundus of these crypts is a thin, single cortical layer, forming the posterior inferior bottom of the maxillary sinus[5]. 4. Permanent maxillary first molar. 5. Deciduous maxillary second molar. 6. Maxillary second premolar. The roots of the unerupted premolars are buccally inclined and therefore project much wider than they actually are. 7. Deciduous maxillary first molar. 8. Maxillary first premolar. 9. Fundus of the crypt of permanent maxillary canine. 10. Deciduous maxillary canine. 11. Permanent maxillary canine. 12. Permanent maxillary lateral incisor. 13. Permanent maxillary central incisor.

# 3.6 The Mandibular Dentition Region

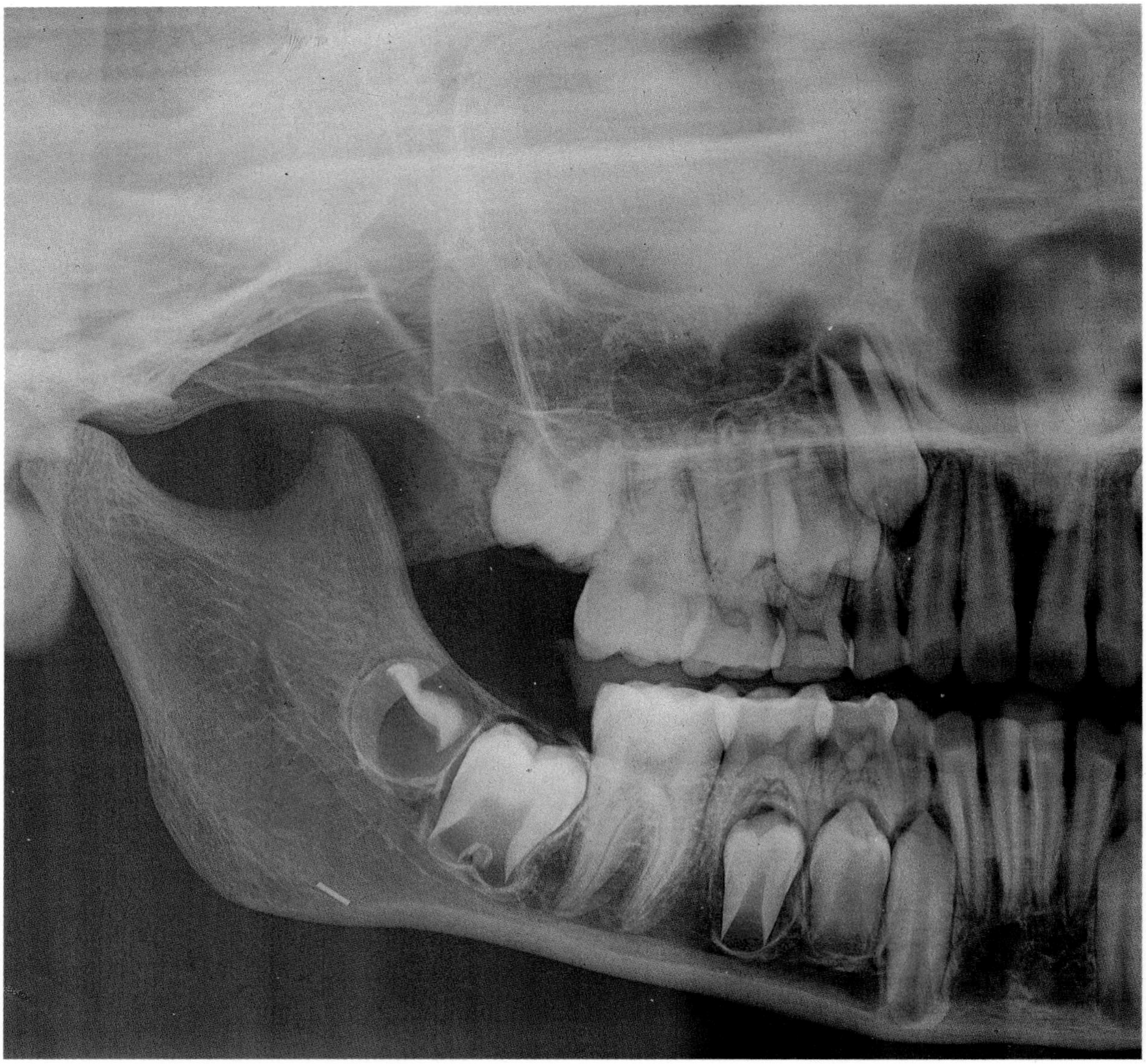

Fig. 57. Right half of panoramic X-ray of dry skull. Mandibular dentition.

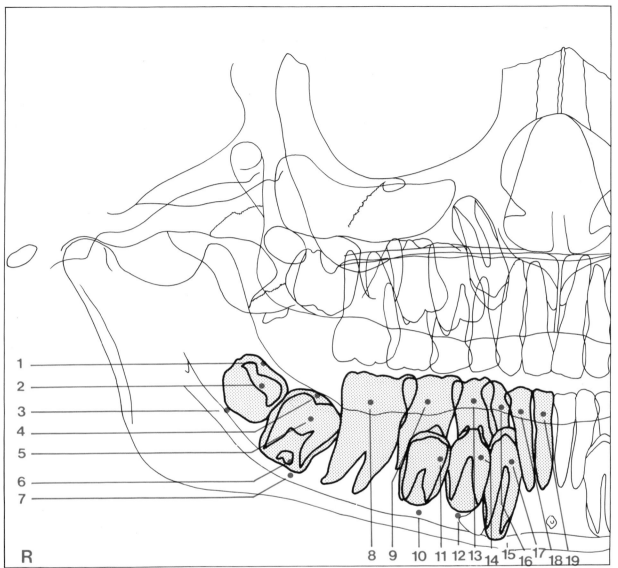

Fig. 58. Drawing of Fig. 57. The mandibular dentition. 1. Roof of the crypt of the mandibular third molar. The crypt is mesially inclined and in the anterior part of the ramus. 2. Developing crown of the mandibular third molar. 3. Fundus of the crypt of the mandibular third molar. 4. Roof of the crypt of the permanent mandibular second molar. 5. The permanent mandibular second molar. 6. The forming bifurcation. 7. The fundus of the crypt of the permanent mandibular second molar. 8. The permanent mandibular molar. 9. Deciduous mandibular second molar. 10. Fundus of crypt of mandibular second premolar. 11. Mandibular second premolar. 12. Fundus of crypt of mandibular first premolar. 13. Deciduous mandibular first molar. 14. Mandibular first premolar. 15. Fundus of crypt of permanent mandibular canine. 16. Deciduous mandibular canine. 17. Permanent mandibular canine. 18. Permanent mandibular lateral incisor. 19. Permanent mandibular central incisor.

Note in Figs. 57 and 59 the difference in the texture of the fundus of the canine and the first and second premolars. The fundus of the canine is still in the cortex of the lower mandibular border, indicating the third stage of crypt formation (see Chapter 4, page 60). The first premolar has started active eruption. Its crypt is in the fourth stage with fine cancellous bone deposition at fundus.

**59**

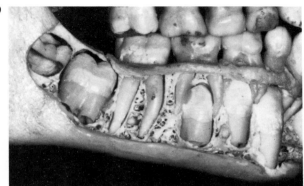

Fig. 59. Lateral view of the mandible of the dry skull of Fig. 57. Note the interradicular bone between the roots of the deciduous molars forming the roof of the crypts of the premolars. Compare the position of the mandibular canine relative to the mandibular cortex with the image seen in Fig. 57.

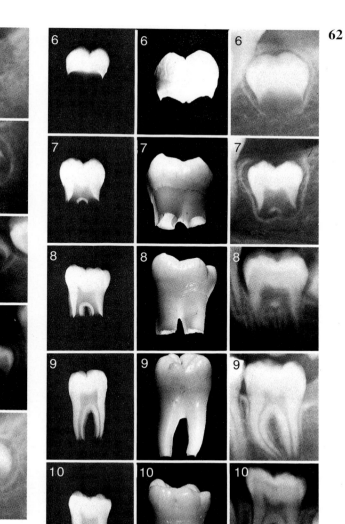

Fig. 62. The 10 stages of development of multi-rooted teeth.

# 4.3 General Aspects of Crypt and Alveolar Socket Formation

This section begins with illustrations that demonstrate, in general, the morphologic features leading to formation both of the crypt and of the alveolar socket that houses the root. Additionally, the developmental characteristics of the buccal region during transition as seen in skulls and in panoramic X-rays are discussed. Finally, changes associated with molar eruption are shown.

The morphogenesis of and subsequent changes in the bone immediately surrounding a developing tooth are directly related to its formation.

Four different stages can be distinguished, each with its own morphology (Figs. 63–66).

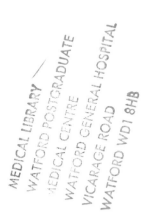

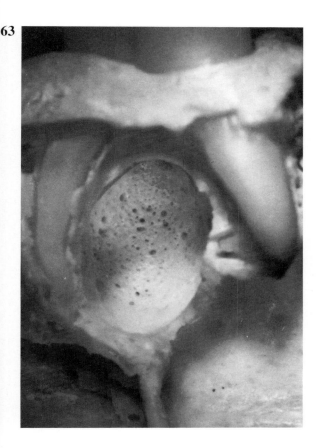

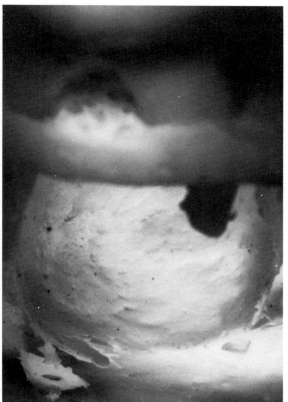

Fig. 63. Crypt formation; first stage.

Fig. 64. Crypt formation; second stage.

The first stage is characterised by formation of the crypt and concomitant crown. All dimensions of a developing tooth bud increase rapidly[37]. This increase corresponds to a rapid increase in crypt dimension through resorption of inner crypt walls and deposition at the endosteal outer crypt walls. At this stage the crypt wall is composed of porous, fine, cancellous bone. In X-rays, only the translucency is apparent, and the wall usually cannot be seen.

Commencement of the second stage is marked by completion of the crown. Remodelling of the crypt walls continues, but more slowly. The original fine cancellous bone increases in density. The extent of compacting and thickening of the crypt walls depends largely on the amount of time available to form the crypt wall. If time is short and development hasty, as, for instance, in the formation of deciduous teeth, porous, fine, cancellous bone is present. Thicker, denser walls are formed during permanent canine, premolar, and permanent molar development. The fundus remains a rather stable area that does not change its relative spatial position until active eruption begins. The crypt wall is very clearly seen in X-rays taken during this stage.

Figures 63 and 64 reprinted with permission from F.P.G.M. van der Linden and H.S. Duterloo, *Development of the human dentition — an atlas.* Hagerstown: Harper and Row, 1976.

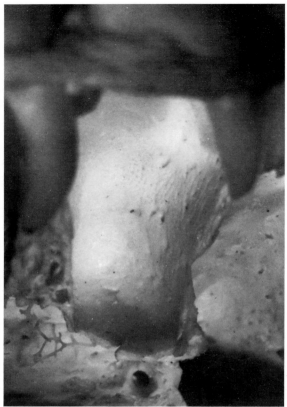

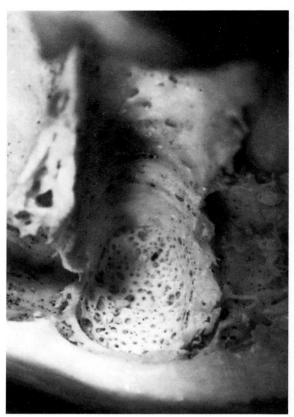

Fig. 65. Crypt formation; third stage.

Fig. 66. Crypt formation; fourth stage.

Crypt formation, third stage begins with the initiation of root development. The surface opposite the occlusal surface of the crown, especially the area around the gubernacular canal (see Fig. 71), becomes resorptive[15]. Deposition of bone takes place around the root to support the tooth. In this stage the initial periodontal membrane evolves. At the fundus there is still no new bone formation. Aspects of the phenomena described above can be seen in X-rays.

This stage is characterised by active eruption of the tooth; fine cancellous bone is deposited at the fundus. Bone deposition at the fundus is followed by a reconstruction of bone in that region. The original walls and fundus disappear in the reorganisation process. The final alveolar socket is then formed by bone deposits around the root, narrowing the space for the periodontal membrane. This stage can be seen very clearly in X-rays.

Figures 65 and 66 reprinted with permission from F.P.G.M. van der Linden and H.S. Duterloo. *Development of the human dentition — an atlas.* Hagerstown: Harper and Row. 1976.

Fig. 67. In this diagram the various characteristics of the erupting tooth and its crypt are schematised as they are seen in X-rays. 1. Resorptive surface at roof of crypt. 2. This part of the crypt is wider, due to resorption to permit passage of the widest part of the crown. 3. Reversal on the bone surface from resorption to deposition. 4. The thickening of the crypt wall here is due to deposition of trabeculae to narrow the periodontal space to support the root. 5. Previously deposition has taken place at the endosteal outer crypt wall surface as the wider part of the crown passed during its eruption. 6. Forming part of the root (Hertwig's epithelial root sheath). 7. The fundus of the crypt. At this stage no deposition occurs; growth in height of the crypt occurs by resorption at the roof. 8. Occlusal surface of the crown. 9. Cementoenamel junction. 10. Developing pulp and pulp chamber.

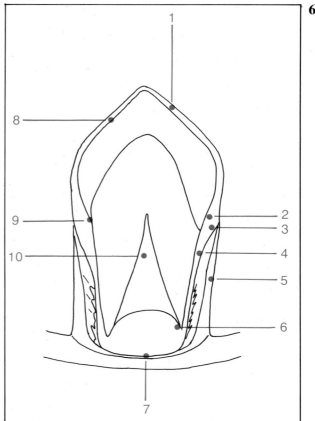

**67**

Figs. 68–73 show bone remodelling of crypts.

Fig. 68. X-ray of part of a dry human mandible; intertransitional stage; permanent canine and premolars in their crypts. The stipple line indicates the plane of sectioning in an upper (Fig. 69) and lower part (Fig. 70) so that roofs and fundus of the crypts can be studied. (×2.)

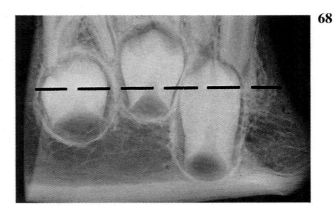

**68**

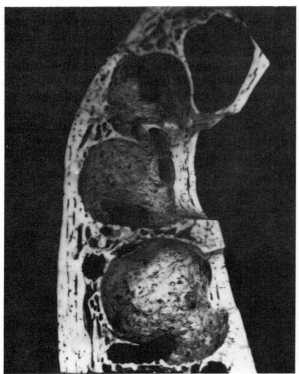

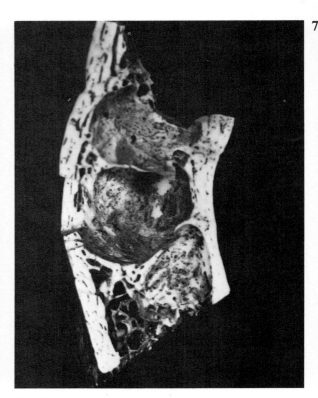

Fig. 69. View at the roofs of the crypt. The large holes are the places where the resorbed root surface of the deciduous teeth were; the small holes are the gubernacular canals. (x3.)

Fig. 70. View at the fundus of the crypts. (x3.)

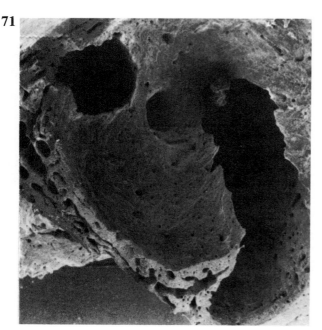

Fig. 71. Scanning electron microscopic (SEM) picture of detail of crypt roof with gubernacular canal. Note the rough surface due to bone resorption by osteoclasts. (x100.)

The description of development of bony crypts and alveolar sockets presented in Figs. 63–73 is brief and simplified; in reality deposition and resorption patterns are much more complicated[5,16,35].

They are affected by the size of the crown in relation to the diameter of the root, and those in multirooted teeth are different to those in single rooted ones. They may also be influenced by the direction of the eruptive movement. When eruption is hindered, deposition in the fundus may change into resorption, and root development progresses then in a downward direction (see Chapter 7, page 118). Sometimes teeth penetrate the dense lamellar buccal cortex during their eruptive movement; sometimes they cause local remodelling changes in the

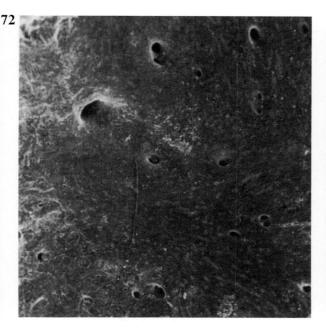

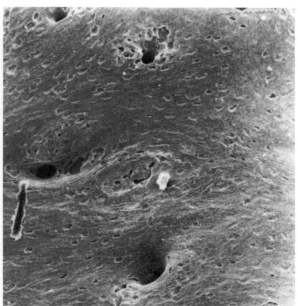

Fig. 72. SEM detail of the fundus of a crypt. Note the smooth surface, indicating a resting surface. (x100.)

Fig. 73. SEM detail of the sidewall of a crypt where deposition is taking place. Note the difference in the bone surfaces of Figs. 71–73. (x100.)

cortex. Some parts of the original socket walls remain as part of the trabeculae that connect

the tooth socket with the buccal and lingual cortex after eruption.

# 4.3.1 The Development of Alveolar Bone

The development of alveolar bone and that of teeth are interdependent in many ways. Alveolar bone develops as a result of direct inductive stimulus originating with the dental primordia[23]. The secondary nature of alveolar bone, expressed by its dependence on the presence of teeth, is, of course, a long established clinical finding.

At the same time, however, the fixation of the teeth in the jaws depends on the supporting function of alveolar bone. The bone of the jaws is of dual nature[13,19]. The *basal* bone develops first in the maxillary and mandibular processus; the alveolar bone forms separately around tooth buds and then unites with the basal bone. This dual origin causes fundamental differences in stimulus/response characteristics between basal and alveolar bone.

During the complex process of development of the dentition[78], alveolar bone undergoes profound changes. Periods of rapid structural remodelling in local areas are followed by periods of slower change and growth.

Bone formation, bone resorption, and then new formation interchange frequently[4]. These changes in alveolar bone are, in part, directly related to the development, growth, eruption, and emergence of individual teeth[15,16]. It appears as if during development each tooth builds its own crypt and alveolus. When a deciduous tooth is resorbed and shed, its alveolus is resorbed as well: this can be seen on X-rays. A new alveolus is formed by the erupting successor. Alveolar bone always remains more porous and more intensively vascularised than basal bone[13]. This makes alveolar bone more sensitive and reactive to outside influences.

This section pays particular attention to the remodelling changes in bony crypts and sockets that are related to the normal eruption around individual teeth in panoramic X-rays. This is of the utmost clinical importance. Not only can one assess how far the root has formed and when emergence is to be expected on an average statistical basis (3/4 of root formed), but also whether that particular tooth is approaching, or is in, the phase of active eruption. Thus, in clinical work, the developmental status of a tooth can be assessed not only by the amount of root it has formed, but also by careful examination of the bony structures around that developing tooth. In contrast to root formation, the rate of eruption (and in part the direction) seems to be influenced by factors in the immediate environment of the tooth.

Such factors are the presence of a deciduous predecessor, its state of root resorption, and the amount of bone above the occlusal surface of the crown of the permanent tooth. Various abnormal conditions, like ankylosis of deciduous predecessor, abnormal position, scar tissue, supernumerary teeth, small odontomas, or follicular cysts may profoundly affect the progress of eruption. It is frequently possible to observe concomitant abnormal bone remodelling changes in such cases.

Representative illustrations of normal development will demonstrate these phenomena in the following section. The clinician can use the principles shown to evaluate progress of individual tooth development in clinical cases. Abnormal conditions are dealt with in Chapter 8.

# 4.4  Alveolar Remodelling as seen on Panoramic X-rays

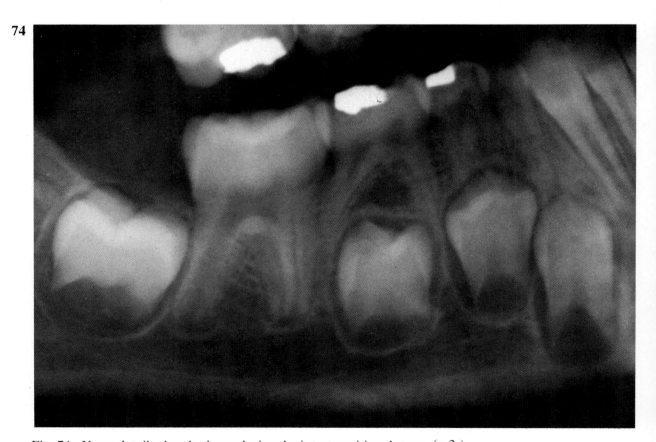

Fig. 74.  X-ray detail: alveolar bone during the intertransitional stage. (x 2.)

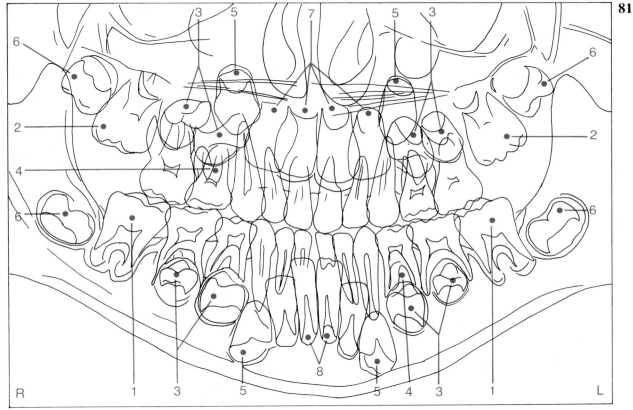

Fig. 81. Drawing of Fig. 80. This is a late deciduous dentition. 1. The permanent mandibular first molars have partly erupted and emerged. 2. The permanent maxillary first molars are still unerupted. 3. The permanent second premolar crowns are partly formed; those of the first premolars are slightly advanced. 4. There is considerable bone present between the roots of the deciduous molars. 5. The permanent canine crowns develop further away from the occlusal level. The upper canines are located laterally to the apertura piriformis, and the lower ones at the mandibular cortex. 6. The crowns of the permanent second molars are partly formed, and as yet no signs of third molar development are visible. 7. The forming part of the roots of the permanent central and lateral incisors is located directly under the nasal apertura. Note resorption at the roots of the deciduous maxillary central incisors. 8. The permanent lower central incisors have begun to erupt. Note the difference in position relative to the laterals. Note also the considerable root resorption at the deciduous central incisors and the lack of observable resorption at the lateral deciduous incisors. The permanent lateral incisors are imaged larger due to their lingual position in the jaws.

Figs. 82-85 show complete deciduous dentition; they are drawings of a skull with buccal alveolar cortex removed.

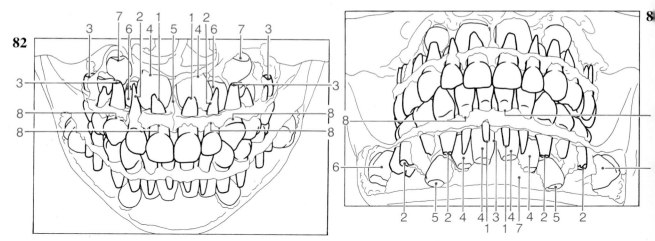

Fig. 82. Frontal view from superior. 1. Marked resorption is found at the apices of the deciduous upper central incisors. 2. The resorption of the deciduous upper lateral incisors occurs mainly on the palatal surfaces corresponding to the adjacent position of the crowns of the permanent central incisors. 3. The roots of the deciduous canines and molars are not yet complete. 4. The forming parts of the crowns of the permanent upper central incisors are situated just below the nasal floor. 5. The bony septum between the permanent upper central crowns with the intermaxillary suture. 6. The mesial halves of the crowns of the permanent upper lateral incisors are located palatally to the central ones. 7. The crowns of the upper permanent canines are situated buccally. Note that the crowns are about half formed and are located just below the orbits and lateral to the nasal cavity. 8. In the incisor region large areas at the cervical border of the deciduous roots are no longer covered by bone (compare with the canine roots). This indicates periosteal resorption and lowering of the crest height at the frontal region.

Fig. 83. Frontal view from inferior. 1. Resorption is found at the roots of the deciduous lower central incisors. Note that more resorption is seen at the root of the right deciduous central incisor than at the left due to the rotated and more labial position of the permanent lower right central crown. 2. As in the upper jaw, the roots of the deciduous canines and molars are not yet completed. 3. The crowns of the permanent lower incisors are in contact with each other; there is no bony separation between them. 4. The not-yet-completed crowns of the permanent incisors are placed in an overlapping position lingual to the roots of the deciduous predecessors. 5. The forming crowns of the lower permanent canines are rather close to the mandibular border and buccally situated. 6. The crowns of the first permanent molars are almost completely formed. 7. The crowns of the permanent lower incisors are situated some distance from the mandibular border. Note that no compact bone is present between the mandibular border and the bony structure just below the forming incisor crowns. 8. Periosteal resorption is occurring at the crest of the incisors but not, as yet, at the crest of the buccal teeth.

Figures 82 and 83 reprinted with permission from F.P.G.M. van der Linden and H.S. Duterloo, *Development of the human dentition—an atlas*. Hagerstown: Harper and Row, 1976.

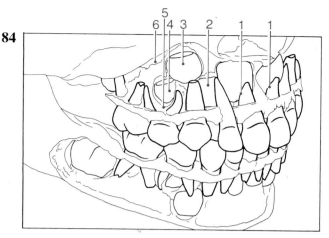

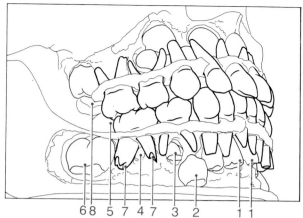

Fig. 84. Lateral view from superior. 1. The roots of the deciduous upper central incisors resorb in an oblique way corresponding to their relationship with their successors. 2. The permanent upper lateral incisor is forming occlusally and lingually to the central incisor. 3. The permanent upper canine is situated furthest from the occlusal plane and located laterally to the apertura piriformis. Note the bony structure at the fundus of the canine, indicating a rather stable situation. 4. The crown of the upper first premolar is about half formed and situated between the roots of the deciduous molar at the apical region. 5. Note the bone at the bifurcation between the roots of the deciduous molar and its successors. 6. Part of the floor of the small maxillary sinus.

Fig. 85. Lateral view from inferior. 1. The crowns of the permanent lower incisors are lingual to the roots of their predecessors; however, they extend buccally to the cervical area. The amount of buccal extension is probably related to the space available and the size of the bony chin button. 2. The permanent lower canine crown is distal to its predecessor and, in this case, situated under the mesial root of the first deciduous molar. 3. The partly calcified first premolar crown with its forming part at the level of the apices of the deciduous molar. 4. The open area where the crypt of the second premolar was located. Note the typical anatomy of the deciduous molar, as described above. 5. The distal surfaces of the upper and lower deciduous molars are in a favourable mesiodistal relationship with regard to the future occlusion of the unerupted first permanent molars. 6. The crown of the permanent lower first molar is complete and situated partially in the ramus. 7. The roots of the second deciduous molars are not yet completed. 8. The alveolar bone at the occlusal surface of the permanent upper first molar is resorbed.

Figures 84 and 85 reprinted with permission from F.P.G.M. van der Linden and H.S. Duterloo, *Development of the human dentition—an atlas*. Hagerstown: Harper and Row, 1976.

# 5.4 The First Transitional Stage

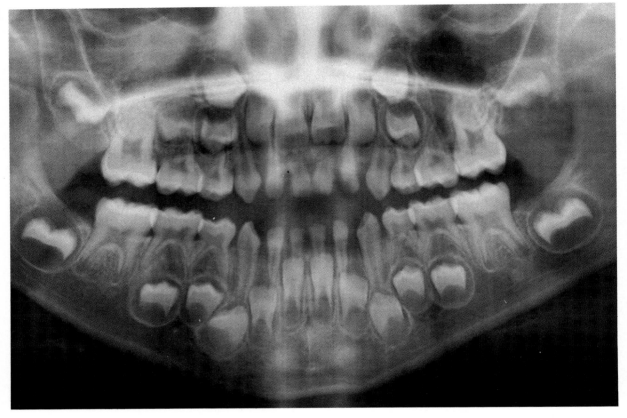

Fig. 86. Panoramic X-ray of the early first transition stage. The indication for taking this panoramic X-ray was the suspected development of Class III with a family history of agenesis of several teeth, and the prospect of interceptive dentofacial orthopaedic therapy.

This stage is characterised by:

1. Eruption and emergence of the first permanent molars.
2. Shedding of the deciduous incisors.
3. Eruption and emergence of the permanent incisors.

It takes about two years to complete this stage. There is relatively little variation in sequence of events. However, a four-year range of variation exists in timing of eruption. Boys are two to four months later than girls.

For the child, its parents, and the dentist this is a most important series of events.

Frequently the clinician is consulted about size and position of the new teeth. Careful clinical intraoral inspection with palpation of the gums is essential. Only in exceptional situations is it necessary to take X-rays of this development. Diastemata are usually normal. Inclination and position of the incisors improve spontaneously, but other factors may form the signs of developing malocclusion. Consult van der Linden and Duterloo, 1976[78]. This first transition stage is demonstrated with three representative X-rays: early, intermediate, and final. In addition, two series of dry skull drawings of the early and final stages are shown.

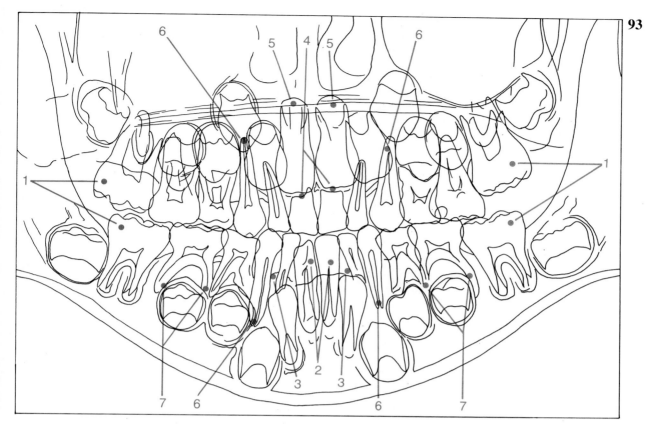

Fig. 93. Drawing of Fig. 92. 1. The permanent maxillary first molars are approaching the occlusal surface; the permanent mandibular first molars are fully erupted; their root formation is about 3/4 completed. 2. The permanent mandibular central incisors have erupted, and their deciduous predecessors have been lost. 3. Note the breakdown of the alveolar support and root resorption at the deciduous mandibular lateral incisors. The permanent lateral incisors have not started their fast eruptive movement. 4. The roots of the deciduous maxillary central incisors are almost completely resorbed, while the same is not true for the roots of the deciduous maxillary lateral incisors. 5. The maxillary permanent incisors are all still located directly under the nasal apertura, though root formation at the centrals is much further advanced. The laterals are imaged larger because of their normal lingual position. 6. The roots of the deciduous maxillary and mandibular canines are fully formed. 7. The crowns of the premolars are at the apices of the deciduous molars.

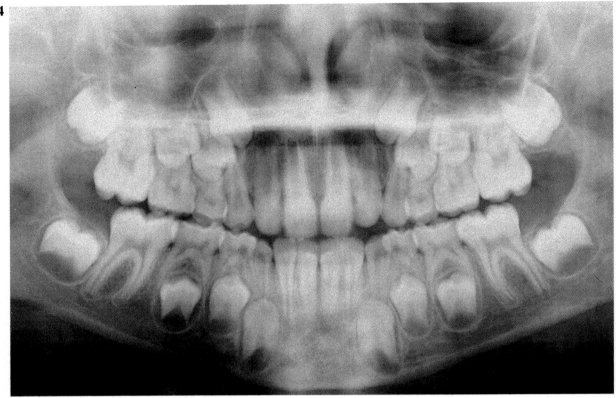

Fig. 94. Panoramic X-ray: completion of first transitional stage.

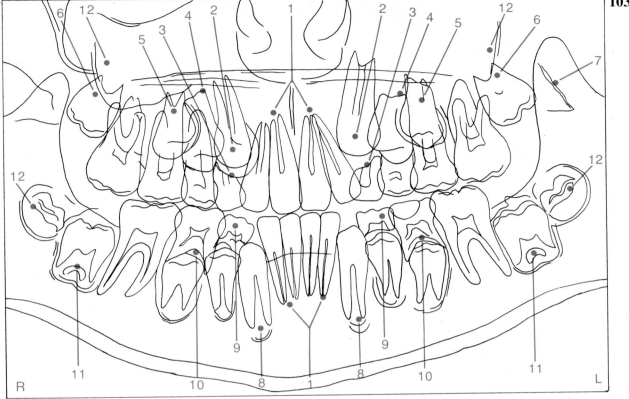

Fig. 103. Drawing of Fig. 102. 1. The apices of the permanent incisors are almost completed. Note the lack of diastemata, the distoinclination of the lateral incisors, and their close relation to the crowns of the permanent canines. 2. The permanent maxillary canines are actively erupting; about 3/4 of their roots are formed. Note that there appears to be no bone present at the distal surface of the root of the lateral incisors. This is a normal feature during this stage, and should not be seen as pathologic. With the eruption of the canines the alveolar bone will form. 3. Maxillary deciduous canine roots are almost completely resorbed. 4. Root formation in the maxillary first premolars is about half. The palatal root, however, of the deciduous first molar is still long. Emergence of the premolar will take another 12 months. 5. The maxillary second premolars have not started active eruption. The roof of the crypt is still visible. The distobuccal and palatal roots of the deciduous second molars are visible. 6. Root formation of the permanent maxillary second molars is about 1/4, and the bifurcation is forming. Active eruption has not yet occurred; the fundus of the crypt is visible as a thin opaque line. 7. Sutura pterygo palatina is accidentally sharply imaged and projected over the coronoid process of the mandible together with the medial and lateral plates of the pterygoid process. 8. The permanent mandibular canines are actively erupting and emerging. The deciduous canines are lost. Rapid bone deposition occurs at the fundus of the crypts. Compare with the fundus of crypts of the premolars. The formative parts are no longer located at the mandibular cortex. 9. The deciduous mandibular first molars are almost completely resorbed, and they appear no longer to have any dentoalveolar attachment. The mandibular first premolars will soon start active eruption. 10. There is still bone present between the roots of the second deciduous molar. At the left side the gubernacular opening is visible. This canal extends from the roof of the crypt to the lingual alveolar crest of the deciduous molar[78]. 11. The bifurcation of the permanent mandibular second molars is forming; root formation is about half complete. 12. It is uncertain whether maxillary third molars will form; they can be present but not yet visible, as variation in timing is very wide for this tooth. The mandibular third molars are at the crown formation stage.

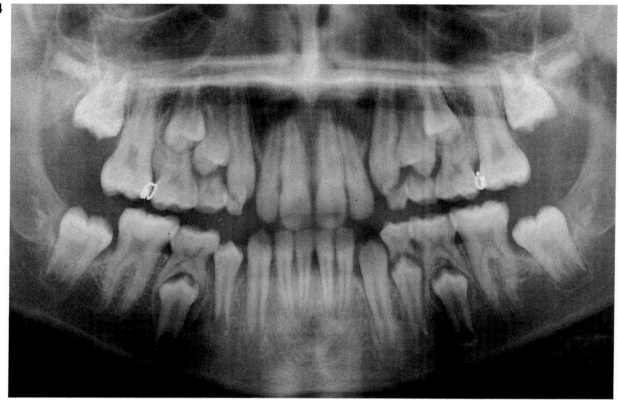

Fig. 104. Panoramic X-ray: second transitional stage—intermediate.

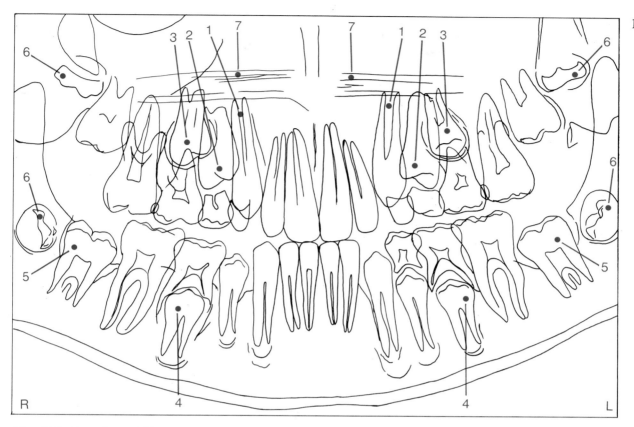

Fig. 105. Drawing of Fig. 104. 1. The permanent maxillary canines are actively erupting; only a small shadow of the crown of the deciduous canines is present. 2. The same is true of the maxillary and mandibular first premolars. 3. The permanent maxillary second premolars are still far from erupting, and considerable root resorption in the second deciduous molars has yet to occur. 4. The mandibular second premolars are more developed than the maxillary ones; there is no longer bone present at the roof of the crypts, but these teeth have not yet started active eruption: the fundus is depicted as a sharp line. Compare with the neighbouring first premolars and canines. 5. The second permanent molars have about 3/4 of the root formed. Note the enlargement of the follicle and accompanying bone resorption. There is no bone seen on the occlusal surfaces, and it will not be long before these teeth pierce the gums. 6. The mandibular third molars appear less developed than the maxillary. Their position is to be considered normal. 7. Ghost images of the hard palate (see section 2.2.2, page 16).

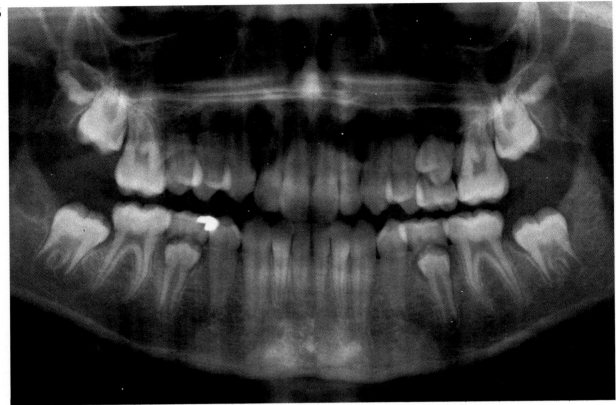

Fig. 106. Panoramic X-rays: second transitional stage, final.

Table 2. Emergence in years of permanent teeth in boys.

| Maxilla Tooth | Very early -2SD | Early -1SD | Average X | Late +1SD | Very late +2SD | Mandible Tooth | Very early -2SD | Early -1SD | Average X | Late +1SD | Very late +2SD |
|---|---|---|---|---|---|---|---|---|---|---|---|
| 1 | 5.72 | 6.46 | 7.2 | 7.94 | 8.68 | 1 | 4.88 | 5.54 | 6.20 | 6.86 | 7.52 |
| 2 | 6.46 | 7.33 | 8.2 | 9.07 | 9.94 | 2 | 5.60 | 6.50 | 7.40 | 8.3 | 9.2 |
| 3 | 9.08 | 10.29 | 11.5 | 12.71 | 13.92 | 3 | 8.34 | 9.47 | 10.60 | 11.73 | 12.86 |
| 4 | 7.68 | 9.14 | 10.6 | 12.06 | 13.52 | 4 | 7.74 | 9.22 | 10.70 | 12.18 | 13.66 |
| 5 | 8.46 | 9.93 | 11.4 | 12.87 | 14.34 | 5 | 8.62 | 10.06 | 11.50 | 12.94 | 14.38 |
| 6 | 4.88 | 5.59 | 6.3 | 7.01 | 7.72 | 6 | 4.84 | 5.52 | 6.20 | 6.88 | 7.56 |
| 7 | 9.88 | 11.14 | 12.4 | 13.66 | 14.92 | 7 | 9.3 | 10.60 | 11.90 | 13.2 | 14.5 |

Table 3. Emergence in years of permanent teeth in girls. Ages are indicated in years/decimals. Adapted from: S. Helm and B. Seidler[33].

| Maxilla Tooth | Very early -2SD | Early -1SD | Average X | Late +1SD | Very late +2SD | Mandible Tooth | Very early -2SD | Early -1SD | Average X | Late +1SD | Very late +2SD |
|---|---|---|---|---|---|---|---|---|---|---|---|
| 1 | 5.60 | 6.30 | 7.0 | 7.70 | 8.4 | 1 | 4.66 | 5.33 | 6.0 | 6.67 | 7.34 |
| 2 | 6.0 | 6.90 | 7.8 | 8.70 | 9.6 | 2 | 5.52 | 6.31 | 7.1 | 7.89 | 8.68 |
| 3 | 8.30 | 9.55 | 10.8 | 12.05 | 13.3 | 3 | 7.5 | 8.55 | 9.6 | 10.65 | 11.7 |
| 4 | 7.54 | 8.82 | 10.1 | 11.38 | 12.66 | 4 | 7.4 | 8.7 | 10.0 | 11.30 | 12.6 |
| 5 | 8.16 | 9.58 | 11.0 | 12.42 | 13.84 | 5 | 8.14 | 9.57 | 11.0 | 12.43 | 13.86 |
| 6 | 4.76 | 5.43 | 6.1 | 6.77 | 7.44 | 6 | 4.78 | 5.39 | 6.0 | 6.61 | 7.22 |
| 7 | 9.46 | 10.68 | 11.9 | 13.12 | 14.34 | 7 | 8.98 | 10.19 | 11.4 | 12.61 | 13.82 |

The estimation of tooth formation age can be determined from four selected teeth.

From birth to 9 years old, permanent mandibular right first molar, first premolar, and permanent canine and permanent maxillary right central incisor are used.

From 10 years old onwards: permanent mandibular second molar, first premolar, permanent canine, permanent maxillary right canine.

The average of the estimated stages is calculated as the formation age and compared to chronological age.

Comparable tables are present in: F.P.G.M. van der Linden, H. Boersma and B. Prahl-Andersen[63].

The actual values for ±2 SD and ±1 SD are used in Tables 2 and 3. Thus, for example, if the maxillary canine is late in a boy aged 14.0 years, one goes to the third row left, where one finds 13.92 as the average value plus two standard deviations. One may conclude that the canine is indeed exceptionally late in emergence because at that age at least 97% of boys have their maxillary canines present in the mouth.

The reader's attention is directed to the large age range, about five years, for teeth emerging in the second transitional stage. For teeth emerging during the first transitional stage this range is about three years.

Table 4. Developmental chronology for the human permanent dentition. Originally based on data of Logan & Kronfeld[46]. The values for the "crown completed" and "apex closed" stages have been modified, according to Haavikko[31].

| Tooth | | Hard tissue formation begins (months/ years) | | Crown completed (years) | Eruption (years) | Apex closed (years) |
|---|---|---|---|---|---|---|
| Maxillary | Central incisor | 3-4 | months | 3.5 | 7-8 | 9-10 |
| | Lateral incisor | 10-12 | months | 4.5 | 8-9 | 10-11 |
| | Canine | 4-5 | months | 4.5 | 11-12 | 13-15 |
| | First premolar | 1.5-1.8 | years | 6.5 | 10-11 | 12-13 |
| | Second premolar | 2-2.3 | years | 7.0 | 10-12 | 12-14 |
| | First molar | At birth | | 3.5 | 6-7 | 9-10 |
| | Second molar | 2.5-3 | years | 7.0 | 12-13 | 14-16 |
| | Third molar | 7-9 | years | 13.0 | 17-21 | 18-25 |
| Mandibular | Central incisor | 3-4 | months | 3.0 | 6-7 | 8-9 |
| | Lateral incisor | 3-4 | months | 3.5 | 7-8 | 9-10 |
| | Canine | 4-5 | months | 4.5 | 9-10 | 12-14 |
| | First premolar | 1.3-2 | years | 5.5 | 10-12 | 12-13 |
| | Second premolar | 2.3-2.5 | years | 7.0 | 11-12 | 13-14 |
| | First molar | At birth | | 3.5 | 6-7 | 9-10 |
| | Second molar | 2.5-3 | years | 7.0 | 17-21 | 14-15 |
| | Third molar | 8-10 | years | 13.5 | 17-21 | 18-25 |

# 5.9 Concluding Remarks

The development of the human dentition, even if no obvious abnormalities occur, is characterised by a large variation in timing. This variation increases with the progress of maturation, which makes prediction of timing of an event unreliable for clinical purposes. The development and eruption of permanent third molars is particularly difficult to predict. Many factors not closely related to tooth development, like jaw size and shape, appear to have difficult-to-measure influences[64-70].

Extensive research on third molars has not yet resulted in useful data for assessment and prediction of events in the individual clinical case. Longitudinal observation might be indicated, and this is the task of every dentist supervising the dental development of adolescents and young adults.

It is recommended that a thorough clinical intraoral examination with *palpation* of the areas where third molars are formed should first be undertaken, before a panoramic X-ray. The predictive potential of the X-ray is limited.

For a review consult F.P.G.M. van der Linden, *Problems and procedures in dentofacial orthopaedics[81]*. Chicago: Quintessenz, 1989[80].

# 6. Interpretation of Position of Permanent Teeth

## 6.1 Introduction

In panoramic X-rays the diagnosis of normal or abnormal position of a tooth in a developing dentition requires thorough knowledge of the normal topographical anatomical conditions of the development stages, and also of the specific manner in which the panoramic X-ray machine produces the image. To help the clinician in this area is the purpose of this chapter.

The dry skull and dentition shown in Chapter 3 are used for reconstructions. This allows close observation of the effects of overlap of complex osseous structures and deciduous and permanent teeth. The spatial relationships of the unerupted teeth and how they are seen in a panoramic X-ray are also shown in these reconstructions. Finally, some frequently seen abnormal tooth positions are created in the reconstructions and compared with the normal situation.

## 6.2 Reconstruction with Erupted Teeth

Fig. 110. Photograph of the reconstruction with the erupted teeth of the skull of Chapter 2. Note the spreading of the buccal and palatal roots of the deciduous and permanent maxillary molars. The roots of the mandibular molars are laterally inclined. An acrylic occlusal splint was prepared to place the teeth in position. Then the splint with teeth was placed in the craniostat (Chapter 2, pages 16 and 17) and X-rayed in standard position.

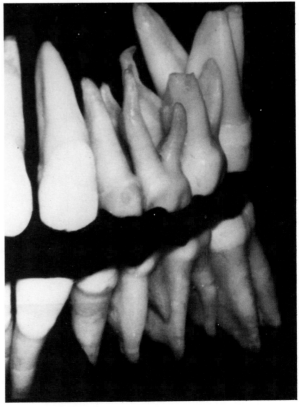

**110**

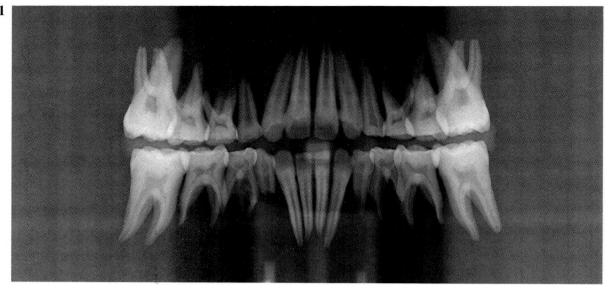

Fig. 111.  Panoramic X-ray of reconstruction with erupted teeth.

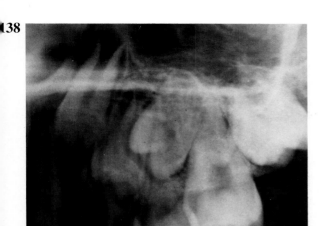

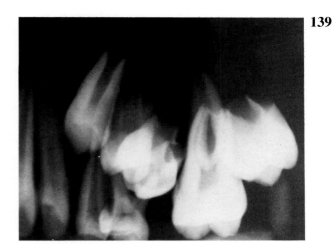

Figs. 138–141. Simulation of impaction of second premolar and mesially drifted permanent first molar. The second deciduous molar is removed.

Fig. 141 shows a view of reconstruction from the apical. Note the rotated first molar.

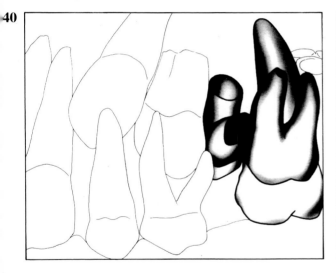

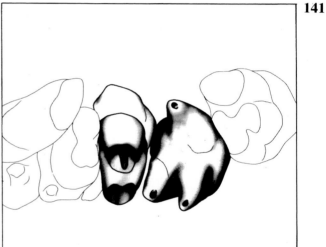

**142** 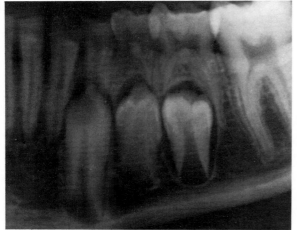 **14**

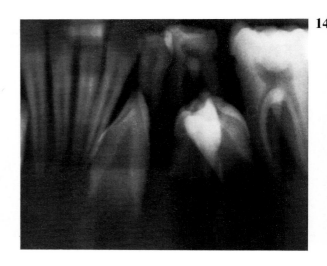

**144**

Figs. 142–144. Simulation of impaction of mandibular second premolar, mesially drifted permanent first molar, and related permanent canine. The deciduous second molar is removed. Note the overlap due to lack of space.

# 6.7 Concluding Remarks

The permanent dentition develops in a crowded position within the jaws. In panoramic X-rays, this usually causes much overlap of structures. Good insight into the normal topographical situations in the stages of development is a prerequisite for correct interpretation of panoramic X-rays of clinical cases.

# 7 Evaluation of Space Conditions and Growth Changes

## 7.1 Introduction

For evaluation of space conditions in a developing dentition, measurements and other procedures should be undertaken. Measuring in panoramic X-rays is seriously limited by lack of standardisation. These limitations have become obvious from the information presented in Chapter 2. It is, however, still possible to extract useful longitudinal information on growth changes from panoramic X-rays of the same individual. Here again, though, limitations are present, and the information obtained should be regarded as additional to or confirmative of information derived from intraoral examination, analysis of dental casts, and cephalograms.

This chapter explores possibilities of evaluation of space conditions and growth changes in panoramic X-rays, with instructive examples. Explanations will be offered as to why certain dimensions are measured on the X-rays and certain special procedures are used. Suggestions for superpositions of serial tracings are also given.

Though only natural developmental growth changes are discussed in this chapter, it should be understood that the procedures could also be used in analysing growth and/or change resulting from treatment.

## 7.2 Evaluation of Space Conditions

The growth of the jaws is frequently insufficient to provide all developing teeth with a place in a harmonious dental arch. Thus, the evaluation of space conditions for the developing dentition is a very important clinical procedure. Discrepancies between arch length needed (which is equal to the total sum of the mesiodistal dimensions) versus the arch length available (the expected length of the tooth bearing area of the jaws) form a key point in diagnosis.

In mixed dentition cases, analysis of space conditions for the frontal teeth and successional teeth can be performed with acceptable accuracy on dental casts and with deduction from tables available for dimensions of the unerupted premolars and canines. However, the accessional teeth are not counted in such an analysis. Space problems for unerupted permanent molars are relatively frequently seen. This cannot be analysed from dental casts, but panoramic X-rays are helpful.

# 7.2.1 Space for Frontal Teeth

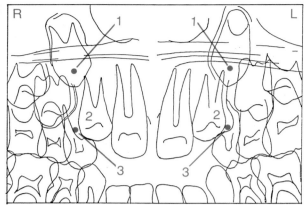

**145**

Fig. 145. Space problems in the frontal region. 1. Permanent maxillary canines; crown formation completed, root formation has started. 2. Permanent lateral incisors are not yet erupted. 3. Extensive root resorption has occurred in the deciduous canines in relation to the eruptive movement and position of the lateral incisor.

Panoramic X-rays, preferably combined with analysis of dental casts, can provide insight into space problems to be expected in the front. Note, in this example, Fig. 145, that there is a small central diastema; the permanent lateral incisors (unerupted) are in contact with the centrals, and have also caused considerable premature resorption of the deciduous canine roots. One may conclude that a space problem is to be expected.

For a reliable evaluation of tooth position, tooth sizes, and space condition in the frontal region, the panoramic X-ray should be analysed, together with the dental cast. Palpation and measurement comparisons of cast and X-ray should provide reliable information. If abnormalities are seen or suspected, specific extra X-rays might be indicated, for instance an occlusal X-ray taken at 60° to the occlusal plane.

# 8.4.1  Premature Resorption of Deciduous Teeth

Resorption and loss of the deciduous canines unilaterally or on both sides occurs occasionally with the eruption of lateral incisors in the maxilla as well as in the mandible. This is usually a sign of space problems (primary crowding). In unilateral situations, one may consider extracting the remaining deciduous canine to prevent aggravation of midline deviation. Premature loss of deciduous canines usually leads to additional loss of arch length, thus increasing the possibility of crowding and malocclusion. Premature loss due to caries may cause severe disturbances of transition and occlusal development.

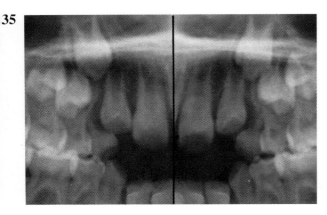

Fig. 235. X-ray detail; premature resorption of deciduous canines; girl 7.8 years old.

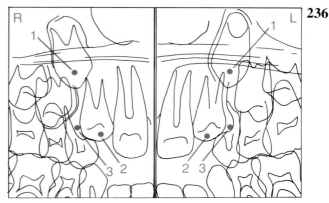

Fig. 236. Drawing of Fig. 235. 1. Permanent maxillary canines; crown formation completed, root formation has started. 2. Permanent lateral incisors are not yet erupted. 3. Extensive root resorption has occurred in the deciduous canines in relation to the eruptive movement and position of the lateral incisor.

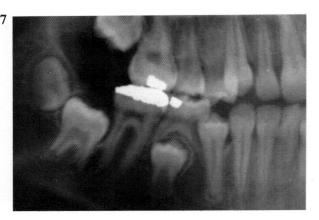

Fig. 237. X-ray detail. First premolar resorbs second deciduous molar; girl 11.3 years old.

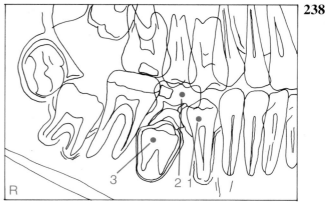

Fig. 238. Drawing of Fig. 237. 1. First premolar cannot erupt properly and has partly resorbed the second deciduous molar. 2. Partly resorbed deciduous molar. 3. Forming second premolar.

# 8.4.2 Prolonged Retention of Deciduous Teeth

This is usually related to trauma or ankylosis. Traumatic damage to deciduous incisors may lead to ankylosis and prolonged retention. Ankylosis of deciduous molars is frequently seen. Four examples illustrate the clinical problems. Usually surgical and orthodontic intervention is necessary.

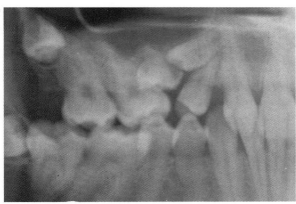

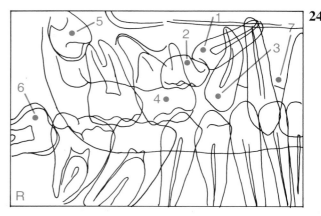

Fig. 239. X-ray detail; girl 20 years old. Ankylosis of deciduous maxillary second molar. It has apparently caused impaction of the second premolar. The crown of the deciduous molar remained in its ankylosed position while the permanent first molar and first premolar erupted and tipped in the diastema.

Fig. 240. Drawing of Fig. 239. 1. Impacted second premolar. 2. Ankylosed—without roots—second deciduous molar. 3. First premolar. 4. First permanent molar, tipped mesially. 5. Impacted maxillary third molar. 6. Horizontally impacted mandibular third molar. 7. Agenesis of lateral incisor.

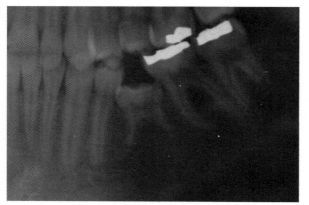

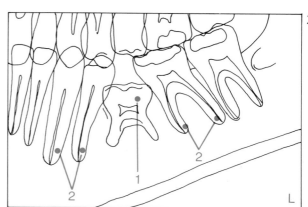

Fig. 241. X-ray detail; girl 18 years old. Ankylosis and infraocclusion of deciduous second molar.

Fig. 242. Drawing of Fig. 241. 1. Ankylosed deciduous second molar. Note the unclear periodontal space. There is agenesis of the second premolar. 2. Relatively long roots are present.

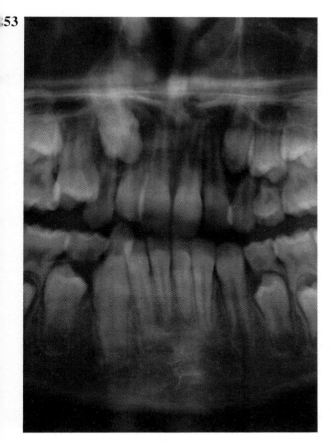

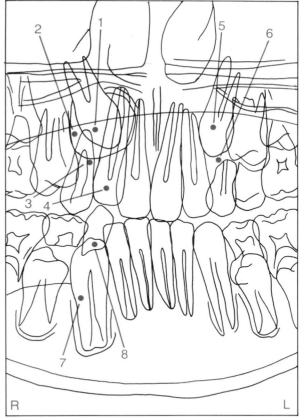

Fig. 253. X-ray detail; girl 11.2 years old.

Fig. 254. Drawing of Fig. 253. Unilateral palatal impaction of maxillary canine and lingual position of mandibular canine. 1. Palatally positioned right permanent maxillary canine. 2. Note the greatly enlarged follicle. 3. No or little root resorption at right deciduous canine. 4. Right permanent lateral incisor appears unaffected. 5. The left permanent maxillary canine is in normal position. Note the size difference of the image compared to the impacted right canine. 6. Root resorption of left deciduous canine. Compare to right deciduous canine. 7. The mandibular right permanent canine has not yet emerged; it is in lingual position. Compare to left canine. 8. Right deciduous canine, largely resorbed root.

In the case of Figs. 253/254, the right canine was not palpable at the buccal mucosa. It had caused a notable swelling at the hard palate. The left canine was palpable at the buccal mucosa. The right mandibular canine was palpable at the lingual mucosa. This mandibular canine erupted without surgical intervention. The right maxillary canine was surgically exposed and a bracket attached for orthodontic traction.

Figs. 255–260 show longitudinal supervision with unexpected impaction of canine.

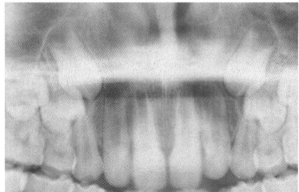

Fig. 255. X-ray detail; boy 9.9 years old.

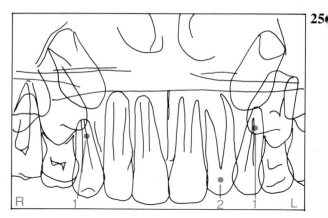

Fig. 256. Drawing of Fig. 255. Normal position of unerupted permanent canines. No differences in palpation. 1. There is a slight difference in root resorption between right and left deciduous canines. 2. Left lateral incisor is slightly rotated.

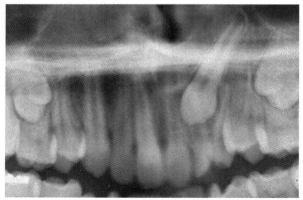

Fig. 257. X-ray detail. Same boy at 13.8 years old.

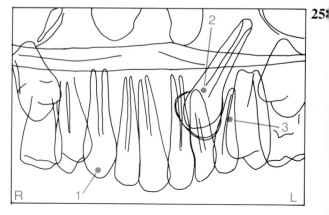

Fig. 258. Drawing of Fig. 257. 1. Right canine: normal eruption. 2. Left canine palatally impacted. 3. No root resorption at deciduous canine.

# 8.7.4  Periapical Resorption as a Late Effect of Trauma

Extensive periapical resorption of alveolar bone may occur after periodontal trauma. Regular X-ray survey of traumatised teeth is recommended.

Fears of losing the traumatised tooth (or teeth) after initial successful attempts to save it are frequently the reason for prolonged re-tention, with, ultimately, loss of the tooth and extensive bone resorption.

In the young child it appears far better that a decision for an integral treatment plan, inclu-ding possibly orthodontic measures, be made. The possibilities for autogenous transplanta-tion of premolars should always be explored.

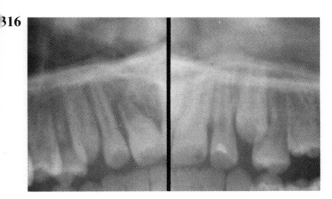

Fig. 316. X-ray detail (Panorex); boy 10.9 years old.

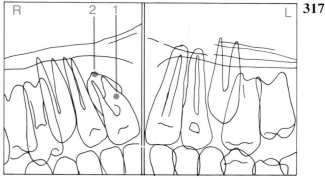

Fig. 317. Drawing of Fig. 316. Luxation of right permanent maxillary incisor at age 6.5. 1. Short root due to termination of formation after pulpal death. 2. Extensive bone resorption. When the boy was first seen, at 10.9 years old, dentitional devel-opment was too advanced to make premolar trans-plantation a realistic option.

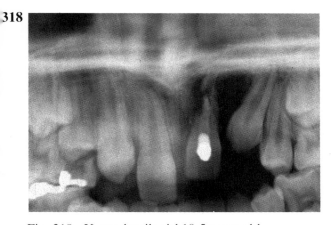

Fig. 318.  X-ray detail; girl 10.5 years old.

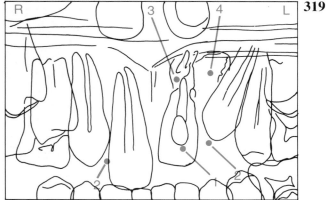

Fig. 319.  Failure of replantation leads to extensive root and bone resorption and chronic infections. 1. Replanted left permanent maxillary incisor, two years after accidental avulsion and replantation. 2. Permanent lateral incisors were congenitally absent. 3. Extensive resorptive destruction of root surface. 4. Large resorption of alveolar bone. See the remark above.

# 8.9 Cysts of Dental Origin

Enlargement of follicle is rather commonly found in developing dentitions. There is considerable variation in the size of follicle around erupting teeth, possibly related to obstruction of eruptive movement. If the translucency is clearly defined, and follicle thickness (in panoramic films) is about 3 mm or more, it is probable that a follicular cyst with epithelial lining is present[6]. If a pericoronal cortex is visible, cyst growth is slow; if not, a rapidly growing condition might be present.

Periapical cysts are seldom found in young children and adolescents. They result from pulpal necrosis and slow loss of periapical lamina dura and trabeculae. The cyst is then seen as a well-defined translucency around the root apex.

## 8.9.1 Normal Follicular Space

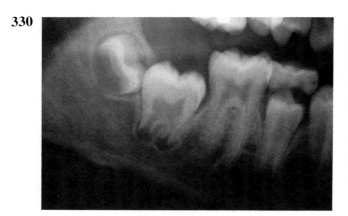

Fig. 330. X-ray detail; boy 12.8 years old.

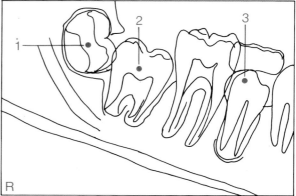

Fig. 331. Drawing of Fig. 330. *Normal follicular space* is seen as a translucency around the developing crown of the unerupted third molar. There is quite some variation in the size of the normal follicular space, particularly in the latest phase before emergence, as is seen in the erupting second molar. Also, the translucency seen around the crown of the second premolar is normal. 1. Third molar. 2. Second molar. 3. Second premolar.

# 8.9.2 Follicular Cysts

The follicular space is enlarged and sharply delineated by a radiopaque lining.

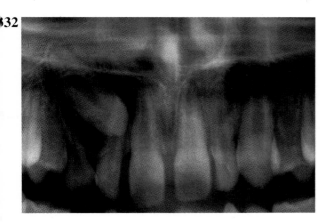

Fig. 332. X-ray detail; boy 13.2 years old.

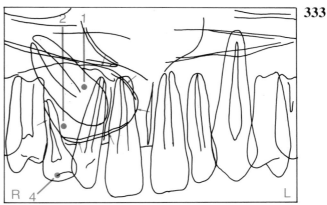

Fig. 333. Drawing of Fig. 332. Follicular cyst around impacted maxillary canine. 1. Palatally impacted permanent canine. 2. Follicular cyst translucency. 3. Radiopaque lining (arrows). 4. Persistent deciduous canine.

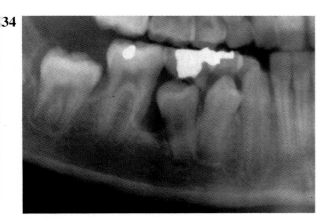

Fig. 334. X-ray detail; girl 10.5 years old.

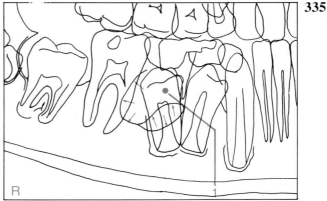

Fig. 335. Drawing of Fig. 334. Follicular cyst around second premolar. 1. Mandibular second premolar. 2. Follicular cyst around crown (arrows). A hard swelling was palpable under the buccal mucosa.

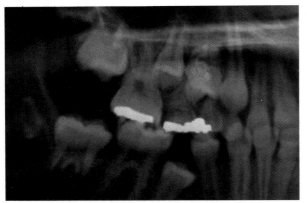

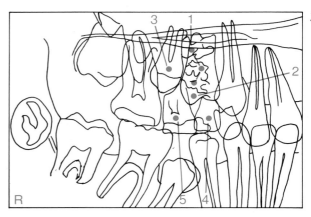

Fig. 344. X-ray detail; girl 9.7 years old.

Fig. 345. Drawing of Fig. 344. Complex odontoma. 1. Mass of radiopaque material. 2. Overlapping unerupted first premolar. 3. Second premolar. 4. Deciduous first molar; resorbed root. 5. Deciduous second molar; resorbed root. A slight hard swelling was palpable at the palate.

# 8.11 Concluding Remarks

This survey of abnormalities in developing dentition is by no means complete.

In the area of congenital deformation and syndromes, there exist many other anomalies not mentioned in this chapter. It is beyond the scope of this book even to attempt to be complete. The purpose is to show the most common conditions, seen on panoramic X-rays.

A similar observation could be made of the section on cysts and neoplasms. Several other abnormalities of these types can be found in children with developing dentitions.

For descriptions the reader should consult oral pathology reference texts[74].

# 9 Abnormalities of the Facial Skeleton and Soft Tissues

## 9.1 Introduction

The purpose of this chapter is to present some abnormalities of the facial structures as seen on panoramic X-rays of the developing dentition.

It is emphasised again that these X-rays were not specifically made to study these abnormalities. Other techniques are more suitable for the evaluation of developmental deformities of the craniofacial region. Standardised lateral and posteroanterior cephalograms, CT scanning, and computer-aided three dimensional reconstructions may be needed. The panoramic X-ray, however, can provide useful additional information.

The chapter is divided into three sections. Each section covers a region of the panoramic X-ray according to the systematic analysis presented in Chapter 3. The three regions are the nasomaxillary, the mandibular, and the temporomandibular joint regions.

As in the previous chapter, it is not the intention even to try to present all possible abnormalities of this vast area. Commonly seen abnormalities, however, are presented, along with some developmental deformities of the jaws that profoundly interfere with the development of the dentition, and which are particularly well depicted in panoramic X-rays.

## 9.2 Abnormalities of the Nasomaxillary Region

### 9.2.1 The Nasal Cavity and Septum

Deviations of the nasal septum are frequently seen, but the part of the septum that is in the image layer and sharply seen is usually difficult to localise anteroposteriorly. Abnormalities of the septum and conchae as seen on panoramic X-rays may give a lead to further examinations or consultations of the ENT and other specialists. Severely deviant septum and conchae are frequently seen in relation to clefts, as the following illustrations will show.

### 9.2.2 Cleft Lip, Jaw and Palate

Panoramic X-rays of cases with cleft lip, jaw and palate show the disturbed morphology of the maxillary dentition, usually very clearly. However, all the limitations that have already been discussed regarding the image of maxillary structures (Chapter 3) are added to the abnormal situation. Nevertheless, the panoramic X-ray is useful to evaluate which teeth are present in the jaws and in which positions.

After that, specific dental films, occlusals, and, if necessary, polytomographic scans can be made to evaluate position and periodontal status of teeth in the cleft region and the size of the bony defects.

Abnormalities frequently seen in these cases are agenesis, supernumeraries or gemination, positional disturbances, disturbances in eruption and eruptive path, and abnormalities in

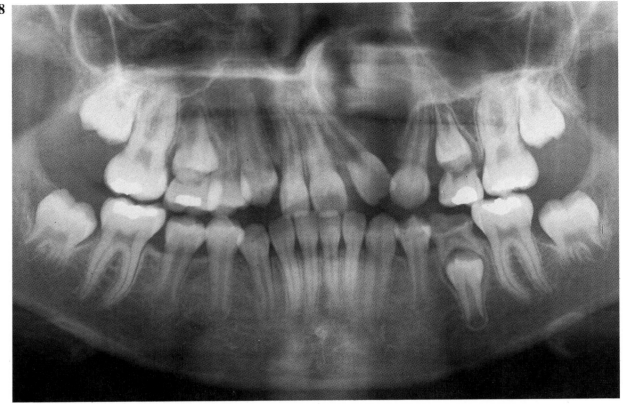

Fig. 348. Panoramic X-ray; girl 12.4 years old.

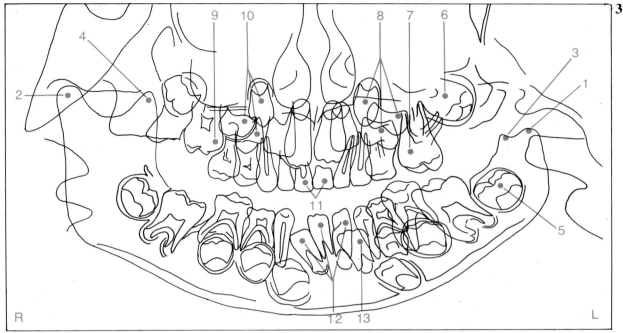

Fig. 390. Drawing of Fig. 389. Hemifacial microsomia. Beginning of first transitional stage. 1. Condylar process left side is absent. There is no joint. Note also the abnormal structures of the fossa and cranial base and compare to normal right side. 2. Normal condyle, right side. 3. Slight indication of a left-sided coronoid process. 4. Coronoid process, right side. 5. Developing crown of left permanent mandibular second molar. 6. Developing crown of left permanent maxillary second molar (dystopic). 7. Mesially positioned and rotated permanent maxillary first molar. The deciduous maxillary second molar has been lost. 8. Unerupted permanent maxillary canine, first and second premolar. 9. Right permanent maxillary first molar is mesially positioned (dystopic) and has partly resorbed the deciduous second molar. 10. Right permanent maxillary canine, first and second premolar. 11. The deciduous central incisors are largely resorbed. 12. Three permanent mandibular incisors have emerged. 13. Left permanent mandibular lateral incisor in lingual position. Note that all left mandibular teeth incline to right as a result of the mandibular asymmetry.

There is severe facial asymmetry in such cases.

Extensive plastic surgical intervention supp-orted by special dentofacial and orthodontic therapy is installed for these patients[32].

# 9.4.3 Effects of Trauma on Further Development

Trauma to the temporomandibular joints in early childhood may lead to growth disturbances, even in cases where no fracture and other pathology (intraarticular haemorrhage, etc.) have been diagnosed immediately after the impact. The effect on further development is probably very variable.

Fractures of the condylar neck may lead to asymmetrical jaw and face growth. It is beyond the scope of the present book to discuss all possible long-term effects of trauma to the jaws during childhood.

The case presented here is an example of long-term effects on further development.

Figs. 391–394 show a girl 10.5 years old.

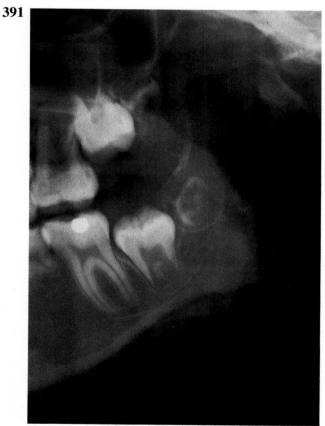

Fig. 391. X-ray, left temporomandibular joint region.

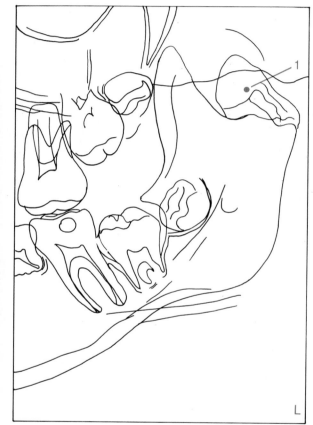

Fig. 392. Drawing of Fig. 391. Fracture of condylar neck. 1. Fractured and displaced condyle.

The fracture occurred approximately three months before the X-ray was taken, and was not diagnosed earlier.

*Angle Orthod* 1980;**50**:121–8.

69. Richardson E.R., Malhotra S.K., Semenya K. Longitudinal study of three views of mandibular third molar eruption in males. *Am J Orthod* 1984;**86**:119–29.

70. Richardson M.E. Lower third molar space. *Angle Orthod* 1987;**57**:155–61.

71. Rönning O., Väliaho M.L. Involvement of the facial skeleton in juvenile rheumatoid arthritis. *Ann de Radiologie* 1975;**18**:347–454.

72. Scheffer M.K. De afbeelding van het caput mandibulae op het orthopantomogram. *Ned Tijdschrift Tandheelkunde* 1984;**91**:397–401.

73. Schultze C. *Anomalien und Miszbildungen der Menschlichen Zähne.* Berlin: Quintessenz, 1987.

74. Shafer W.G., Hine M.K., Levy B.M. *A textbook of oral pathology.* 3rd ed. Philadelphia: W.B. Saunders, 1974.

75. Tammisalo E.H. Professor Yrjö V. Paatero. The pioneer of panoramic oral tomography. *Dent-Max-Fac Radiol* 1975;**4**:53.

76. Ten Cate A.R. *Oral histology: development, structure and function.* 2nd ed. St Louis: C.V. Mosby, 1985.

77. Thilander B., Rönning O., eds. *Introduction to orthodontics.* Stockholm: Tandläkarförlaget, 1985.

78. van der Linden F.P.G.M., Duterloo H.S. *Development of the human dentition—an atlas.* Hagerstown: Harper and Row, 1976.

79. van der Linden F.P.G.M. Models in the development of the human dentition. In: McNamara Jr. J.A., ed. *The biology of occlusal development.* Monograph 7. Ann Arbor, Michigan: Center for Human Growth and Development, 1979: 43-60.

80. van der Linden F.P.G.M. *Development of the dentition.* Chicago: Quintessenz, 1983.

81. van der Linden F.P.G.M. *Problems and procedures in dentofacial orthopaedics.* Chicago: Quintessenz, 1989.

82. Volk A. Uber die Häufigkeit des Vorkommens von fehlenden Zahnanlagen. *Schweiz Monatschr Zahnhkd* 1963;**73**:320–34.

83. Welander U., McDavid W., Tronje G. Theory of rotational panoramic radiography. In: Langland O., Langlais R.P., Morris C.R. *Principles and practice of panoramic radiology.* Philadelphia: W.B. Saunders, 1982.

# Index